A Doctor's Quick Way
to Achieve Lasting Beauty

A Doctor's Quick Way to Achieve Lasting Beauty

"How to Play the Beauty Game"

ROBERT ALAN FRANKLYN, M.D.

and

MARCIA BORIE

Published by
INFORMATION, INCORPORATED
NEW YORK, NEW YORK

Copyright © 1970 by
Robert Alan Franklyn, M.D.
All rights reserved

. . . There's only one corner of the Universe you can be certain of improving, and that's your own self. So you have to begin there, not outside, not on other people. That comes afterwards, when you have worked on your own corner . . .

—ALDOUS HUXLEY

Contents

Foreword: The Game of Life

PART I:
LIFE IS A GAME—PLAY IT!

Chapter:
1. The Game of Life
2. Playing Post Office
3. The Game of Hide and Seek
4. The Game of Tug of War

PART II:
LIFE HAS OBSTACLES—CONQUER THEM!
5. Hollywood Beauty Tips
6. General Beauty Quiz
7. The Do's and Don'ts of Beauty

PART III:
LIFE IS A MYSTERY—SOLVE IT!
8. The History and Mystery of Scent
9. How's Your Aura?
10. Play the Beauty Game: Psych & Scent
    Your Man!
11. The Sweet Scent of Success

PART IV:
LIFE IS A CHALLENGE—MEET IT!
12. The Good Life
13. The "Durable Dynamo Diet"
14. "T = T & T"
15. Only Thirty Days to Go!
16. More Quick Ways to Achieve Lasting Beauty
17. "Fad and Fantasy" Diets
18. Weight Stabilizing Recipes

PART V:
LIFE IS A BATTLE—WIN IT!
19. Exercises—American Style
20. Yoga and You
21. Spice Up Your Life

PART VI:
LIFE IS A GIFT—TAKE IT!
22. The Beauty Pavilion
23. Breastplasty
24. Banish Wrinkles in a Wink!
25. To Wig or not to Wig? What a Question!
26. The Shampoo
27. Sun Fun
28. Massage: Rub-a-Dub-Dub
29. Stand up to Beauty: Your Feet, Hands,
        Eyes & Ears

PART VII:
LIFE IS A GLORIOUS ADVENTURE—
        TRY IT!
30. Do-It-Yourself Cosmetics

PART VIII:
LIFE IS KNOWLEDGE—GAIN IT!
31. Basic Beauty Encyclopedia
    Epilogue

Part I

Life Is a Game—Play It!

*Three grand essentials to happiness
in this life are something to do,
something to love, something to
hope for.*

—JOSEPH ADDISON

The Game of Life

Strictly speaking, life is a game . . . a game of chance . . .
a coming together of two sets of genes which result in
human creation . . .

You are a product of this most fundamental game. The
question is: What kind of a product are you?

We hope this book will inspire you to take a look
at yourself, honestly, and to improve those areas which
need improving.

Are you still chronologically young? Are you a post
deb? Is yours an emerging personality, or are you already
a fully formed adult?

Do you have a career? Is it personally rewarding?

Are you a housewife struggling to find a few minutes
for yourself in each busy day?

Are you single? Divorced? A middle-aged woman
still looking for love?

Whatever your state in life at the moment, more than
likely it is safe to assume you would like to change places
with someone else . . . Look like someone else . . . Act like
someone else . . . Turn the clock back and begin again.

Why? Because the human animal is rarely satisfied . . .

The whole point of this book is to enable you to face reality. *You are you*—that cannot change. Why get bogged down with self-defeating thoughts of what might have been?

Today, you CAN work on the you that is until you become the you of your dreams.

How? Quite simply, by first ridding yourself of fears, doubts and unhappiness. Does that sound like pure pablum? Well, it isn't!

The point, dear ladies, is that enough time and tears are wasted in frustration to generate the power needed to move Mount Everest.

Well, we're not interested in moving mountains. What we are concerned with is moving every individual closer to her ideal goals.

How? By simply letting you in on the most advanced, most efficacious ways we know of achieving lasting beauty.

It all begins with your attitude toward yourself. Toward life. Throughout this book you will find literally dozens of methods for self-improvement. Think of each as a game . . . meet each challenge with a determined smile. If at first you don't succeed—learn to laugh at your first attempts—and begin again.

Remember, the more you look upon these routines as burdensome or difficult the less effective they will be, and the less you will accomplish.

But why belabor the point? Let's go to it! PLAY THE BEAUTY GAME and have fun doing it. Don't set impossible goals. Be realistic. But remember—you are playing the game for very high stakes—the prize is a new you to be proud of!

No matter what results you achieve, think of yourself as a winner . . . Never again be plagued by self-defeating despair. Revert to your childhood attitudes toward life.

a game. Keep them in mind and then begin to play—the adult way—with hope and confidence.

Within these pages you will find literally dozens of ways in which you can help yourself—immediately, quickly —to achieve Lasting Beauty. Everything has been designed to show you the shortest, most enjoyable, most rewarding methods for self-help. Take a chance! You have nothing to lose but your bad habits, excess poundage, age-lines, grey hair and unnecessary bulges!

Good luck! Have fun . . . and remember, life is a game . . . a game of chance . . . Take a chance. Be a winner!

Playing
Post Office

Start on the road to achieving lasting beauty by sending yourself a letter. Select your prettiest stationery and begin.

Dear Me . . .

Today, I have embarked on a new way of life. I will be playing a whole series of games with only one participant— me.

I will set my own goals . . . make my own rules . . . follow my own guidelines . . . I will be, at all times, the captain of the team!

Playing games is fun. I will play many games . . . and *I will have fun* because every game I play will lead me one step closer to the me I want to be.

To begin with, I will honestly analyze my face, my body, my mind, my emotions. I will make a list of all my good points. To it, I will add those areas in which I need help. Then, once I know what I need, I will begin to develop a routine which will provide me with solutions to my needs.

I will start immediately because life is a swiftly moving game—and I want to play it! Fully!

Although I realize that other people and events will

6

crowd my schedule, I will nevertheless make time for myself. *Prime time!*

Always, while I am "Playing the Beauty Game," I will keep my sense of humor about it. However, I will not care what others think of me and my games. I will happily proceed unhampered by any outside influences. I will be able to do this because I know the results will be so pleasing that no one who loves me can be offended by my self-involvement.

To be beautiful means to care about me as well as about others . . . To be beautiful means not only giving but partaking . . . To be beautiful means to be loving of others, but first I must love myself.

Sometimes I may seem thoughtless, as inconsiderate as a child . . . but I am not! What I am is an adult who is fully aware of the games I must play in order to be the best possible me.

You see, I want to be beautiful . . . desirable . . . charming . . . self-confident . . . vital . . . I want to be alive— truly alive—in every sense of the word.

I want to be happy . . . content . . . I want to be able to take whatever comes in my stride . . . I want to be strong so I can stand up straight and smile at every day's events . . . I know that there will be times when my heart is heavy, when disappointments fill the moments . . . but if I am beautiful and strong I will bend like a branch in the wind —but I will not topple over. . .

I cannot . . . I will not . . . I must not give way to self-doubt or despair. If I do, the games will be over . . . and I do not wish the games to end—ever!

Today, I have begun to work toward achieving lasting beauty. In order to do this, I must play many games . . . and I *will* be a winner!

Love,
Me

The Game of Hide and Seek

This is a very special game directed at those of you who have lived with obesity for a long period of time.

With some, overweight begins as far back as early childhood. You started out as a plump baby with adorably pinchable cheeks. You grew into a plump child, easy to cuddle, seemingly happy with your extra padding.

In truth, once the realization of your poundage problem hit you, inwardly you were miserable. The other kids teased you, called you names which were funny to them but which made you cringe. In defense, you ate more, kept your hurts to yourself and continued to grow —up and out.

By the time you reached high school, life was, for you, a lousy, unfair game. You felt like a person with one foot in quicksand. Desperately you tried to extricate yourself, but the more you struggled, the deeper you sank.

School dances and social outlets were denied you. Again, in defense, you turned to food for comfort. Now the relatives who chucked you under your adorable plump baby chin were beginning to nag. Really nag. Now when it's too late, well-meaning parents suggest a diet, hide the cookies, threaten, cajole, and finally use the ultimate weapon—SHAME.

"Aren't you ashamed of yourself? All the other girls in your class are so popular. What's wrong with you? How can I take you shopping when nothing we see fits you? Don't you realize boys like girls who are slim and attractive?"

The harsh words of people you love are like nails, coffin nails, and they bury you deeper within yourself. Sometimes, in desperation, you want to cry out: "Please, help me—don't nag me!" But usually the words stick in your throat. Your pride has been deeply wounded. Your self-confidence has been shattered. If even those who love you criticize you, what hope is there?

By the time you are out of high school, the deadly pattern of self-destruction has been finally set. So you live out your life hiding behind loose shifts and tent-size coats, and for you the game of life is, indeed, heartbreaking.

From that point on, the pattern varies. In desperation, you marry a boy—any boy who'll have you—usually a fat one who has known rejection himself. Together you are Mr. and Mrs. Misery.

Or you get a job and stay single and play the martyr . . . the woman who can be counted on to work overtime because she has no place to go . . . no one waiting for her . . . no life beyond the confines of the office.

Okay, so that is the way your life has gone up until now. Today, no one expects anything of you—except maybe to use you as a baby sitter on those evenings when the neighborhood teenager fails to show up!

Today, infected with self-pity, you live each day with no hope, no expectation, no nothing.

If you will read these words and not reach for a hot fudge sundae, then the process of misery can be reversed! If you can honestly face up to all your fears and doubts and disappointments and toss them aside and begin again, then life, for you, can be a beautiful game.

Select one of the diets in this book. See your doctor and get a checkup. Then begin the process of revitalization. Start losing weight. Start experimenting with makeup. Do daily exercises. Treat yourself to facials and beauty baths and every other preparation geared toward self-improvement.

Sometimes, to move quickly, means to pace one's self as a long distance runner does. Don't expect to be a new you in one week. It's taken you years to become what you are. Give yourself a *realistic* amount of time to begin to look beautiful. Meanwhile, keep busy. Stop being the office martyr or the relatives' babysitter! Use your free time for yourself. Begin to like yourself, . . . to care about yourself. Begin to seek every avenue for self-improvement that is available.

All your life you have hidden behind a mound of fat. Take it off. Seek beauty. Never again play the game of just hiding. Instead, play the game of seeking the you that is underneath all the bulk. Remember, don't make your task burdensome. Learn to play the game with hope and happiness in your heart, and you, too, will be a winner!

The Game of
Tug of War

No matter who you are, where you live, how much your income, life may seem to you to be one continual Tug of War. A series of pulls and yanks which lead nowhere.

Well, *that* game is over for you as of right now! No more being pulled and yanked. Today, you begin to play a new game of war. The enemy is yourself. The battleground is life as you have lived it up until now. Your goal is lasting beauty. The method of attack is to PLAY THE BEAUTY GAME for all it's worth!

Beginning right now, you are a field general, deploying the troops, planning the strategy, mapping out the campaigns.

Since it is impossible, in a book written for a mass audience, to cover every single human contingency, we can only give you an idea of how this particular game is played. Then you will be on your own, and if your attitude and action is correct, the victory flag will be yours.

11

We have already discussed the perpetually obese female. Now let us look at the lady who lately has let herself go . . . the woman who has become dependent upon girdles and waist cinchers to keep in those extra few pounds she's put on over the past year or two.

In conjunction with this lady is the woman who used to take great pains with her looks, but who is now disgusted with those age lines and grey hairs and who, in desperation, has decided to grow old prematurely and go to pot as rapidly as possible.

As a Hollywood Beauty Doctor, a plastic surgeon who has dealt with thousands of women, I am firmly convinced that no *healthy* female prefers to be unattractive.

I am positive that the instinctual desire for beauty is within every woman. Everyone of you can be more attractive, younger-looking, more desirable. What's more, once you get that way, you CAN stay that way.

So, be a field general. Evaluate the strength of the enemies which plague you. Plan your strategy employing those games which will solve your individual needs.

Read all the chapters of this book. Then go back to the beginning and start to play those games which will bring you to personal victory.

There is a great deal of glory in being a general, and a large amount of responsibility as well. The success of the campaign is on your shoulders. You can decide to attack and defeat the enemy, or you can blow a bugle and loudly sound a call to retreat. The choice is yours. Take it! Damn those heavy hearts, full spead ahead!

Have fun, general . . . the results of your victory will be like gleaming medals for all to see and admire!

Part II

Life Has Obstacles—
Conquer Them!

*People do not lack strength;
they lack the will . . .*

—VICTOR HUGO

Hollywood
Beauty Tips

No one has more fun "Playing the Beauty Game" than a smart woman whose life-style demands that she "be on display" constantly. With this in mind, we have consulted dozens of international beauties from the jet set and the world of show business. From them, we have collected a whole series of beauty tips and special secrets which will make your own "Beauty Game" easier to play.

Although it may seem otherwise, we can personally assure you that Hollywood's beautiful stars have the SAME basic annoying human problems as those shared by you who read this book. After all, today's screen jet setters and love goddesses were once little flesh and blood girls with the same needs and desires, and ALSO the same figure, hair and skin problems. As a result, today beauty rituals from around the world have been utilized to make debutantes, post debs, and stars the most ravishing creatures on earth.

Herein you will find hints about make-up and skin care. Beauty aids for your hands and feet, your eyes and hair. Read them all. Take those suggestions and tips which suit your own needs best. We can't guarantee you'll marry a prince or win an Academy Award, but the results you WILL receive can be just as valuable to YOU.

"Sunset Strip Contour Straps"

Cut two pieces of cheesecloth about 4 inches wide and long enough to tie or pin over the top of your head. Place one of these cheesecloth strips directly under the chin and tie firmly over the top of the head. Place the other strip farther back about where the chin merges with the throat line and tie over top of head. Saturate the cloths under the chin with an astringent lotion and make icy cold by passing a piece of ice over the cloths. When you remove these bands, after they are dry, you will be amazed at the improvement in your appearance. It is as necessary to use astringents as it is to stimulate circulation and add nourishment, for you must help the skin to retract and at the same time keep it elastic.

Six Basic Skin Types

NORMAL:	An even textured and even toned skin with a young, dewy looking glow.
DRY:	A parched, sometimes lined skin with hard-to-see pores. Usually a chapped texture that prevents make-up from looking natural.
MATURE DRY:	An aging dry skin that shows wrinkles and exaggerated dry skin problems: fre-

quently caused by carelessness . . . lack of previous treatment care . . . or constant exposure to sun and wind.

OILY: A shiny complexion caused by excess secretion, particularly through the center of the face and across the forehead. Enlarged pores, blackheads, and occasional blemishes.

COMBINATION: A complexion that suffers oily skin problems through the center of the face and forehead, and is plagued with dry skin problems around the outer areas.

PROBLEM: A skin disturbed with blemishes and acne-like problems.

There are a quartet of creams women should familiarize themselves with—and then use when necessary:

1. Cleansers (cleansers and skin fresheners)
2. Softeners (bedtime creams or lotions)
3. Stimulants (astringents and masques)
4. Protectors (moisturizers)

Skin Fresheners

Skin fresheners are a mild blending of cleansers, created to rinse away traces of left-over cleansing cream and to leave the skin immaculately clean. Skin freshener is a part of the cleansing process. Its function is to remove the invisible film of cleansing cream residue. This residue holds unwanted waste. If this matter is allowed to stay in the pores, surface roughness may occur. Astringents are intended to tighten the pore openings in order to give a finer texture. This constricting action might seal in unwanted waste if used without a skin freshener.

Stimulants

Basically, stimulants are designed to brighten skin tone and promote the illusion of a fine porcelain-like texture. Stimulants offer another dimension for complexion improvement, that is, an almost immediate lessening of the "fatigue look". By encouraging facial circulation a generally drab tone can be awakened with a glow of youthful radiance. Stimulants applied immediately before make-up application give a vibrant expression that is remarkably lasting. Also, when the skin is smooth, make-up applies easier—and appears more flattering. The smoother the skin, the easier it is to apply and to see the glories of color foundation.

Cleansers

Authorities in the field of cosmetics strongly believe that a woman's complexion is only as good as her cleansers and faithfulness of application. If make-up, grime, and natural skin waste is allowed to remain on the skin, the surface will become rough . . . and treatment creams will be unable to penetrate and do the job intended. Every woman, without exception, needs a liquid or cream cleanser, to reach into tiny pores and whisk away unwanted deposits. When waste matter is allowed to remain in the skin, pores become enlarged . . . and even the healthy function of the skin can be hindered.

Soap and water washing is good enough—if you are not particularly interested in preserving or improving your beauty. Most soaps tend to intensify dry skin problems: Cream cleansers can effectively penetrate the pore openings and gently pamper a complexion. Even the finest soaps cannot reach into tiny pore openings. Soap should be considered for surface cleansing only, for it can only take away a portion of stale make-up. For a superb feeling of freshness, authorities suggest an astringent or skin freshener always be utilized immediately after cream cleansing. The marvelous tingling sensation and feeling of immaculate cleanliness imparted by a facial rinse is delightful to feel, and it gives encouragement for brightening the natural tone of the skin.

Also, you should be sure to cream cleanse your face first thing in the morning even though it has been thoroughly cleansed the night before. This rule applies because while you sleep the facial area secretes waste through the pore openings. If this microscopic discharge is not effectively removed, a surface roughness may occur which eventually results in enlarged pores. Particularly those of you with either oily or combination skins must pay close attention to your morning skin cleansing.

Use of Skin Lotions

Skin lotion products should be used after cleansing and before applying your foundation.

If you purchase the proper skin lotion, it can be a most beneficial beauty aide. If used after an oil-base cleanser, it will serve to remove any traces of grime, excess oil and make-up. It also stimulates circulation and helps to give your skin a fresh, clean look.

Because good skin lotions produce a gentle astringent action, they help to firm and tone your skin. Finally, a good skin lotion minimizes pore openings.

Incidentally, during the day, your powder and foundation shades should be the same color. However, in the evening, your powder should be pinker or one or two shades darker. You see, the evening light tends to cast shadows and reduce the desired liveliness of background make-up.

Protectors

During the day, when skin encounters the elements, temperature changes, and is exposed to the dehumidified atmosphere of steam heat and air conditioning, natural mositure can be drained at an increased rate. Usually the glamorous coverage of make-up *cannot* provide sufficient treatment protection to alleviate this condition. Special moisturizing preparations that can safeguard skin, and at the same time enhance the loveliness of make-up, are vital.

Moisturization is so important because without a proper percentage of moisture in the skin's cells, the overall complexion appearance looks withered, dull, drab and old. Only lotions prepared with readily absorbed moisturizers can affect thirsty cells and help them respond and function normally. At night, while we sleep, the skin reacts most favorably to a rich consistency of emollients balanced with moisturizers. During the day the complexion requires the help of humectants and special protective ingredients . . . because no make-up is a tonic to the skin. It cannot act as a complete protecting agent and a glamorizer at the same time. The addition of moisturizers into a foundation can further enhance the over-all charm of make-up. Regardless of the time of day, or whether or not you wear make-up, the skin should be gently protected with a moisturizing preparation. Contrary to popular opinion, an oily skin needs just as much moisturizing care as any other type skin.

Night Creams

All skin types require bedtime treatment cream. While we sleep, our body performs a "repair job". Our nervous system is refreshed, and muscle tension caused by the previous day's activity is alleviated. While we are unaware of skin fatigue, this vital organ can become weary, too. It needs refreshment. Unfortunately, nature is not always able to replenish necessary moisture and oils at a sufficient rate to keep the skin young looking and beautiful. Be mindful, too, that the aging process begins long before twenty-one, which means the body is no longer able to keep pace with the evaporation of moisture and oils. In the case of oily skin, nature cannot always control excess activity, even though our bodies are at rest. Then, too, oily skin is susceptible to occasional dry patches. Also, oily skin that is neglected tends to become coarse in texture and to develop scale, which is solidified secretion. An oily skin requires moisturizing just as much as a dry skin to assist in restoring the healthy function of the skin cells.

"Spacial Facial Techniques"

1. Cleanse your skin thoroughly.
2. Apply a rich nourishing cream, patting it in gently with the cushions of the fingertips or a rubber patter.
3. Pat with fingertips starting under the chin and continuing until you see the circulation surging to the surface; follow along each jawbone, upward on the neck and along the cheek to the front of the ear on both sides of the face.
4. Pat expression lines from mouth to nose and upward on the forehead from eyebrows to the hair line.

5. NOTE: Be careful—do not stretch the skin with the patting movements.

6. Remove any remaining cream with a tonic lotion and follow with an astringent.

Night-Time Tenderness

Use your favorite night cream, applying it carefully as directed below:

A. Use your left hand on the right side of your throat, and the right hand on the left side of your throat. Make little circles from base of throat to jawbone. Using your hands alternately, stroke gently up center of throat.

B. With the fatted palms of both hands, pat up on your cheeks several times.

C. Lift frown lines with short strokes, using both hands as though "combing" forehead.

D. Starting at outer eye corners and working towards nose, fingertap gently over eyes.

E. Leave on overnight.

Foundation

The beauty of a woman's complexion may often be dependent upon the tint and texture of her foundation. Minor flaws, such as uneven tone and shadows, seem to disappear when a woman applies the appropriate foundation for her skin type—and applies it as directed. Wise selection of color is imperative. At night you should always wear a foundation shade that is darker and more intense in color. Women with sallow skin should apply a pinker color that is also a shade darker than her daytime shade.

Today tinted foundation is a blessing within every

woman's grasp. It can be used to great advantage in creating illusions.

For instance, if your nose is prominent, a shade darker than the usual should be applied to that area only. On the other hand, if your nose is too long a darker foundation shade applied to the tip of the nose will give the illusion of a shorter, more becoming nose. If you want to highlight a facial area, such as the cheekbones, you should apply a lighter than usual foundation shade. Women with round faces, who prefer a more slender appearance, should apply a slightly darker foundation to the outer edge and jaw area.

Face Powder

History has revealed time and time again that face powder was among the earliest cosmetics used by women. Thousands of years ago, women of position considered powder a precious possession. Through the centuries this particular beauty aid has grown in popularity and today still maintains its place as a "must" in the smart woman's cosmetic wardrobe.

With the creation of compressed powder, today's woman has become confused between the distinctive function of loose powder compared with the newer form. Loose face powder should be applied immediately after tinted foundation has been smoothed on and allowed to set for a minute or so. The best way to apply face powder is to pat-press on generously, then allow powder to rest on the skin for a minute and lightly brush away excess. If your skin is oily or your nose has a tendency to become shiny, it is advisable to splash on cold water after the excess powder has been brushed away. Gently pat dry with lightest touches of soft cotton. The time a woman should apply compressed powder is later in the day, or evening, when make-up might require refreshing, or a woman's nose becomes shiny. Usually powders contain a slight amount of foundation and fine powder particles that help restore a fresh make-up look. Cake powder should be smoothed on lightly. Reapply if necessary, but do not rub on.

Lipstick

Of all the cosmetics women apply, lipstick is most affected by changes in fashion, changes of skin tones, and changes of hair coloring. For instance, you are susceptible to changes in skin tone because of almost constant contact with the out-of-doors and with frequent changes in weather. Your hair coloring, influenced by cleanliness, sun and wind contact, as well as purposely by professional color changes, affects the shades of lipstick which are more complimentary. Therefore, as always, you should be prepared. How? By having on your cosmetic table at least three basic shades which go well with the current fashion trends and colors. These three are: coral tints . . . pink tints . . . bright red tints.

The corals go best with warm, vibrant, vivid costumes. Pink tints blend well with cool, serene colors. Bright reds brighten and frame the neutral shades.

Choosing a lipstick or a wardrobe of basic lipstick colors is actually quite a science—a unique formula—well worth learning and then remembering. Lipsticks should not only be influenced by your skin tones, hair and eye coloring, and the clothes you wear, but also by the occasion. When dressing casually for an afternoon business or luncheon date you might choose more natural looking tones within the three basic color groups. For evening, or a more dressy occasion, you then choose

a more intense, dramatic color within the basic group-
ings. Then, too, if your skin is pale or delicate, stick to
a soft, unjarring color. If you have a sallow or olive
complexion, use the lighter shades.

Generally speaking, women with medium brown to
light blonde hair should avoid overly dramatic lipstick
colors. As a rule, ladies with dark brown to brunette
hair will look most attractive with more intense lipstick shades. Women with gray hair may choose either
soft or medium shades, depending on the shade of gray.

Among today's exciting new cosmetic aids are the
frosted or slicker lipsticks. Using either as a topcoat over
your regular lipstick gives you a shimmering, jewel-like
sparkle.

Shape, Don't Drape, Your Lipstick

A pair of lips beautifully curved and filled in with a
luscious color are a joy to look at. Poorly shaped lips
can be improved—the natural lip line *can be* changed.
Defects *can be* eliminated.

1. Your lipstick make-up tools should include a lip
liner brush and at least *two lipstick shades.*

2. The brush is used to outline the lip shape (some
also like to fill in with the brush) using a deeper-toned
lipstick for the outer edges and a lighter-toned lipstick
to fill in the fullness of the lips.

3. Both lipsticks must be in the same color tone of
course. Blue reds used together—yellow reds together,
etc.

4. Before you start, blot lips dry. Keep mouth relaxed
while drawing outline. Hold lip brush as you would a pencil. Steady the hand by placing the little finger firmly on
the chin. Fill the brush with color and start your line.
Outline your upper lip first—then lower lip.

5. Next fill-in outline directly from the tube.

6. For longer lasting results, wait a few moments for the color to set, then blot excess with a tissue.

7. If a richer color effect is desired, apply a second coat of lipstick—and blot again. For moister lips, apply slicker or frosted now. Don't blot.

Quick Tips to Beauty

1. A beautiful face should begin with healthy feet! Why? Because blood circulation in the feet is very important to overall relaxation and good health. Here are some tips for improving *facial* beauty through the feet:

A. Have a good pedicure preceded by a quarter of an hour session with a foot vibrator. Massage feet, ankles, calves and knees with oil heated to a luke-warm temperature (olive oil is good for this purpose).

B. In lieu of a vibrator, massage feet by hand with a good lubricating oil. Follow this with a foot bath. Alternate soaking your feet first in hot water for one minute and then in extremely cold water for one minute. Ten minutes in all. Not only does this make your feet feel great, but the instantaneous healthy glow on your face will amaze you.

2. For a quick, inexpensive facial, buy a small tin of Fuller's Earth at any drug store. Mix it with a quantity of Witch Hazel until it is the consistency of paste. Apply evenly. Let the mixture dry on your face. Wash off with tepid water followed by cool water.

3. To make a do-it-yourself milk bath, fill your tub with hot water and pour in a mixture made of cornstarch and mineral oil (you can substitute a quantity of real milk) until it is the consistency of a thick liquid. For extra luxury sprinkle a few drops of your favorite perfume or bath oil into the tub. Now step in and lie

back, immersing your body as far as possible. In moments tension lessens and you will feel relaxed.

4. For tired, calloused feet, you can try a scented foot bubble bath. Soak feet for 10-15 minutes. Dry. Gently apply a pumice stone to wear away dead skin and callouses. Apply a scented talc or foot lotion. Repeat 3 times a week.

5. Here's a good facial pick-me-up. Beat 2 egg whites until they stiffen. Apply all over face and neck with fingertips. Lie down and relax for 10-15 minutes. You will feel the preparation working as your skin tightens. Wash off with tepid water. Rinse with cold water. You will look and feel glowing.

6. The proper use of make-up can give you the *illusion* of a narrow nose, if you employ a white make-up pencil. Draw a thin line down the center of your nose, then apply your make-up base. Complete the illusion by using a shade of make-up base on each side of the nose, which is darker than the base on your face. If you want to give the nose a shorter look, add a dab of the darker base under the tip of your nose.

7. It is possible to stay cool cosmetically during hot summer days by keeping your lipsticks in the frigidaire. Also keep face lotions and a bottle of your favorite cologne in the ice box—cold lipstick will not become gooey. A cotton pad, saturated with cold astringent to cleanse your face followed by a freshly applied make-up, and set off with a generous supply of icy-cool cologne, will give you that summertime sparkle.

8. For a new wave set sensation try setting your hair with milk. Shampoo and rinse hair carefully. Apply milk (put a quantity in an atomizer bottle for easy application). Comb hair well until milk is evenly distributed and then proceed to set hair as usual. (NOTE: This page out of grandmother's "recipe" book is good

for those with *normal and dry* hair types. Those with oily hair should *not* use this milk set.)

9. For traveling, be sure to pack one of the new skin perfumes or creme sachets which come in non-breakable, non-spillable forms. Your favorite scent is essential to feeling and looking your best while en route.

10. In between combing and spraying your hair use a damp comb run gently through your set to "revive" the spray's holding action.

11. In cold weather most perfume does *not* have quite the same lasting power as usual due to reduced body heat. To stay pleasingly aromatic in winter try using perfumes more frequently, and be sure to reinforce your fragrance throughout the day and evening.

12. Today you *can* have scent from tip to toe—literally! A recently arrived new product on the market—scented nail polish! In tones ranging from very pale pink to hot garden rose, each fragrance is as different as each shade. This interesting polish is quite simple to apply and makes your hands an extra focal point in your over-all total beauty aura.

The polish sets and dries rapidly, releasing a scent of roses or spices. No excuse now not to sparkle and scintillate from head to toe. Use scented polish after your pedicure, too!

13. Here's a good hair conditioner for use after your shampoo. Beat 2 eggs well. Massage into hair. Leave on for 10 minutes. Comb through hair to evenly distribute. Rinse with lukewarm water. Be sure all traces of egg are washed out. Your hair will be lustrous, easier to manage, and noticeably more silky.

14. Under artificial lights color is drained from the skin. Therefore your lipstick should be deeper and bluer in tone. Foundations should have more pink than

beige at night. Eye make-up should be more dramatic and the entire make-up slightly heavier in tone.

15. If you need special attention in the chin area, take a thin terry cloth towel and wring it out in warm water. Twist the towel into a rope and slide it back and forth under the chin, going upward and outward. Be gentle, not brisk; be sure the towel is kept moist.

For special under-eye care, soften an eye cream between your fingers, then pat it on the under-eye area with a "press and lift" motion.

16. If your skin tends to be dry, rich creams should be used often, and should remain on your face longer. Avoid astringents! Don't rub too hard, use only a soft washcloth. Creaming with an emollient is often a solution to the problem of dry skin.

Here are some skin care don'ts.

Don't—apply ice directly to your skin. If you must use ice—as an astringent, for example—first wrap it in a washcloth or towel, otherwise you'll see little red veins appearing on the surface. These are broken blood vessels.

Don't—touch your face unless absolutely necessary. Above all, avoid touching blackheads, whiteheads or other skin blemishes.

Don't—retire without removing all your make-up.

Don't—scowl or grimace. Avoid pulling down the corners of your mouth. Avoid pressing your lips tightly. Such unlovely mannerisms can cause even more unlovely lines.

17. False eyelashes *can* be beautifying if correctly used. The trick, once you've purchased eyelashes, is to put them on (as per directions) and then trim them with a manicure scissors once you have them securely on. Avoid the exaggerated "Minnie Mouse" look by

trimming your lashes so they enhance your natural lashes while not looking excessively fake.

18. Learn to use the new under-foundation blushers now on the market. Blushers are a real boon to every lady who wants to look as pretty as possible. Blushers not only tend to improve your over-all look, but serve as facial contour aides as well. There are several shades on the market. Be sure you test each shade on clean skin and select the proper color.

19. To keep weight down, try eating a dill pickle for dessert instead of something fattening!

20. For dry skins, try frequent applications of coconut oil. You'll be pleasantly surprised at the results!

21. To stay in tip top condition mentally as well as physically, treat yourself to a sauna bath and massage at least once every six weeks. If you can afford it, have a sauna steam and massage several times a month.

22. To give your face a necessary treat, try applying beauty grains at least once a week (depending on skin type). As always, the cleaner your skin, the healthier your complexion will stay!

23. Be sure to keep your lips moist. Even around the house, apply lipstick or at least a covering of lip gloss or glaze every day. Avoid dry, cracked lips as though they were the plague!

24. Before that special evening (and as often as possible, big evening or not) get a short rest in a dark room. Place eye pads moistened with soothing lotion over each eye. Relax. Think happy thoughts. Drift off day-dreaming about how to "Play the Beauty Game" more effectively.

25. To keep fine hair attractive, settle on a short, softly waved style, slightly bouffant for fullness. Avoid too many curls as they tend to make fine hair frizzy. At home, set hair in large pin curls or rollers for a smooth

set. Be sure to have a professional haircut and shaping every five or six weeks. With fine hair, we advise washing it at least once a week (more frequently if oily) to avoid limp look.

26. For dry hair, a good *pre* shampoo conditioner is advised. Follow our directions for a hot oil shampoo at least once every few weeks. Use fat rollers in setting to avoid split ends.

27. To avoid chapped lips, watch out for certain bad habits. *Avoid* moistening mouth before applying lipstick. *Avoid* licking lips and pressing them together to blend lipstick. *Avoid* running your tongue over teeth to remove excess lipstick. These motions frequently keep lubricants from penetrating the skin. For a moist and beautiful mouth, blot lips dry, then try applying one of the new colorless lip glazes that are now on the market. The glaze softens lip surface. Wait thirty seconds and then apply your lipstick. Apply top layer of lip glaze until your lips are once again smooth. If you do not care to apply second coat of glaze, then finish setting lipstick by brushing on a thin coat of translucent powder to set.

General Beauty Quiz

Over the years, these have been the most frequently asked beauty questions. Some of the information in our answers is contained elsewhere throughout the book, but you can't repeat these answers too often!

Is foundation beneficial to the complexion?
Foundation gives protection to the complexion but not to the degree of a moisturizer. A woman should always apply a moisturizer before smoothing on tinted foundation. Actually, the consistency of both preparations is compatible and will enhance the overall beauty of make-up.

Does the type of shampoo used for weekly shampoo affect hair coloring?
If a detergent shampoo is used, the brilliance and natural looking beauty of a hair coloring can be affected up to 25 percent. To avoid this problem, use a

32

shampoo with a creamy formulation which contains cleansing ingredients that will leave the hair miraculously clean but will not affect the color.

Is medicated shampoo drying?
Medicated shampoo retards excess secretion, but does not drain the hair of essential oils.

How can a shampoo benefit my troubled skin?
Science has shown that oily hair attracts and holds dirt because oil is naturally sticky. Also, bacteria of the hair and scalp become enveloped in the excess oil that clings to the hair shaft. This unwanted grime can transfer to the complexion as hair brushes across the face.

My hair is tinted, should I use a creme rinse?
A woman who uses any color change product should never shampoo without following up with a creme rinse. Hair that has been chemically treated is susceptible to dryness. A creme rinse acts to balance this condition.

Will a hair conditioner take the tinted color out of my hair?
No. A good hair conditioner will not disturb the tinted color of the hair but will affect the texture of the hair by creating new softness and brilliance. If hair has been color rinsed, a good hair conditioner plus the application of hot towels for approximately 30 minutes will drastically reduce the unwanted artificial color. If you have used a semi-permanent coloring, and follow the plan described above, a degree of the artificial coloring will be absorbed by the hot towels.

Should I use a hair conditioner before a permanent wave?
All hair types should be treated with a good hair con-

ditioner before a permanent wave. This protects the hair against the abrasive action of permanent wave lotions, which can cause temporary dryness and lack of lustre. Use the conditioner a few days prior to the permanent wave.

Are the hair conditioners on the market recommended for family use?

Definitely. Children and men suffer with dry hair problems just as women do. Children will not object to a hair conditioner treatment as it is quick and neat to apply, requires a few minutes waiting time, and rinses off without difficulty. Discuss the various hair conditioning products for sale with your local cosmetics saleslady. She can help you select the best product for your hair.

Does setting the hair with beer really help?

It depends on your hair. If it's fine and thin, beer may give it some body. If it's oily, beer will help lessen the oil. In general, however, we recommend a good hair setting gel, specifically for your own hair type. There are numerous products of this type on the market to-day.

When I sun on the beach, I wear dark glasses to cut the glare, but I am now developing white rings around my eyes. How can I avoid this?

Try putting small cotton pads saturated with eye lotion over just your lids while you tan the rest of your face.

I'm on the go all day. How can I stay fresh looking? Right now, as the day progresses, I feel as if my lipstick and eye makeup is smeared. Yet it is impossible for me to wash my face during the day. What can I do?

Frankly, we know of no way to get through an entire day and still look fresh without making a few repairs. However, a careful make-up in the morning will help, and if you apply eye make-up over a powder "foundation," it should not smear. Then "set" your make-up with a cotton pad wrung out in iced water or chilled skin lotion (helps keep a fresh look). Press the pad gently over your whole face, concentrating on your nose and chin, which are likely to get most oily. Another idea: Carry a small flat sponge in a small waterproof bag in your handbag and wring it almost dry; remove the shine, but not your make-up, by giving your face a light swipe with the sponge. Apply fresh lipstick. Also, the new facial sprays for setting make-up appear to be quite effective for most skin types.

Is it true permanents don't take on pregnant women?

False. In fact, it's a good idea to have a permanent a few weeks before the baby is scheduled to arrive so your hair will be easy to care for in the hospital and when you get home. Another good idea: have a conditioning treatment for your hair just before the baby is due.

I'm only in my twenties but already I have a double chin, yet I am not overweight. Is there anything I can do about this?

Yes. Even women in their fifties and sixties can maintain a firm chinline. Try throwing you head back as far as you can, open your mouth wide for a moment, and then close it slowly, ending with clenched teeth. Hold for a few seconds, relax and repeat four times. Run through this routine at least five times a day.

What causes hangnails and how can I prevent them

and the rough skin around my nails? I have a baby, and my hands are always in water. Could that be the reason?

Dryness usually causes hangnails and rough skin, and when hands are kept in water a lot, they do dry out. Wear rubber gloves when you must have your hands in water. Use hand cream before and after each dunking, and keep your cuticles tidily trimmed. A professional manicure can get you off to a good start.

I have dark shadows and wrinkles around my eyes— perhaps the result of a recent weight loss. What can I do to make them less apparent?

You should use an eye cream around the clock. In the daytime, you can mix a little of the eye cream with a foundation a little lighter than the one you use on the rest of your face and fingerprint it lightly into the area around your eyes. Blot off any excess with tissue. The lighter foundation will help to conceal shadows, and the eye cream will help to relieve dry skin around your eyes. Persistent bags and wrinkles are easily removed by simple plastic surgery in a few minutes without hospitalization.

I have a big mouth—really a big mouth. Is there any special shade of lipstick that will make it look smaller?

It's not so much the color of your lipstick (except that you should use natural-looking clear-red shades) but how you apply it. Use two lipsticks, one a little lighter than the other. First outline your mouth with a brush dipped in the lighter lipstick, being careful to draw the line just inside the edge of your lips. Fill in with the darker shade.

The Do's and Don'ts of Beauty

Under artificial lights color is drained from the skin. Therefore, your lipstick should be deeper and bluer in tone. Also, foundations should have more pink than beige at night, and your eye make-up should be more dramatic. Here are some other tips to help you look more lovely.

In applying cream rouge, after blending the foundation carefully, apply three tiny dots of rouge (right on the foundation) placing the rouge high on the cheek (never lower than the line of the nose as a rule). Use the tips of the fingers to blend the rouge, always upward and out. Feather off the edges so no line of demarcation shows, and smile into your mirror when you apply the rouge. This shows the high point of the cheek. Blend a little rouge on this curve.

For the Full Face: Place the rouge on the high part of the cheek closer to the nose and blend lightly across the too full area.

If the Face Is Too Slender: Aid the illusion of width by placing rouge on curve of cheek slightly away from the nose and blend out and up to temples.

If the Face Is Square and Heavy Along the Jaw Line: Soften the angles of the jaw line by shadowing. Pat on rouge, then blend down across the square part.

Apply a little rouge to shadow a bony "bump" under the eyebrow.

A soft blending of rouge under jaw line or chin takes away a heavy drooping effect.

In Applying Face Powder: Always use a clean piece of absorbent cotton or puff to apply powder.

Use lots of powder and press (not fluff or pat on) it into the foundation - this aides in *cling* and sets the powder for a longer lasting effect.

Next smooth the puff over forehead down the cheeks and over chin for a satiny finish.

Your compact powder shade should be a little darker than loose powder.

Try a lighter powder over a darker foundation for evening.

In Applying your Foundation: First—Always cleanse the skin and be sure to "rinse" away all surface oiliness. *Second*—Apply a small amount over neck and face until completely satiny dry. *Third*—Apply foundation in dots over cheeks, forehead, nose and chin. Do not use too much. Blend with fingertips until every bit of skin is covered. Carry to ears and hair line and work lightly until completely feathered off and no line shows between skin and foundation.

Beautiful Eyes

Eyes are considered by many "experts" to be the loveliest feature of the face. They "light up" the person-

ality. They can be large, limpid and glowing with reflected color framed by perfectly arched brows and
thick lashes.

To make the most of your eyes, here are some hints:

The eyes should be rinsed daily with a special eye lotion used in an eye cup. Eye lotion is both healing and
soothing and washes the eye free of dust particles, helps
inflamed eyes and keeps the membrane soothed and clean.

Use two shades of pencil—for a brunette, etch the
brows first with brown, then gently emphasize with black.
Blend up and out with an eyebrow brush. Grey (char-
coal) is softer on most brows than black.

The color of eye pencil and mascara should harmonize.
Blue with blue, green with green, etc.

Always make the pencil point very sharp—lines must
just be an illusion very finely drawn.

1. Frame the eyes and make them appear larger. Use the
eye pencil to draw a fine line just above the upper lashes,
making the line thin at inside corner and gradually widen
the line as you near the outside corner. Lift the line slightly
as you finish the corner . . . never let the line drop downward.

2. For a soft line—use eyebrow brush dipped in a little
cream mixed with eye pencil (blend on the back of the
hand) and use the brush to darken the brows. This is very
soft and pretty for older women or for very light coloring.

3. If the brows are thin—brush the eye pencil through
the hairs the wrong way (towards the nose) then use the
eyebrow brush and brush the brows up and out. This
darkens each little hair and there is no harsh line against
the skin.

4. To tweeze eyebrows—it is best not to do this, unless
necessary. Use a magnifying mirror. Tweeze slightly above
and under brow and over bridge of nose. Never tweeze
too much and never make the natural brow into a thin
line.

5. Unruly brows may be controlled by a bit of hair-spray or wave-set lotion applied with eyebrow brush.

Eye Shadow

Eye shadow is one of the loveliest of the entire make-up bag of tricks. Its use makes the eye more luminous, more mysterious, larger and more deeply colorful. Matching the color of the iris deepens the color of the eye itself. Then, letting the imagination run riot, the use of eye shadow colors can transform the "orbs of the soul" by completely changing their color, elongating or rounding the shape of the eye, shadowing too prominent bone formations, or highlighting sunken eyes.

For general use, apply eye shadow on the lower part of the lid close to the upper lashes. Blend the color from corner to corner. Use only a little dot of color and blend with fingertip or brush the color on with a soft camel's hair brush.

If the eyes are heavy-lidded, blend shadow over the entire lid and right up the brow—blend off softly.

If the eyes are deep set or too close together, blend shadow from center of eye out to corner.

If the eyes are spaced too far apart, blend shadow close to nose corner and stop at the center.

Use brown shadow on puffy eyelids to set back a "bony" upper part of eye.

Use a soft background eye shadow first and blend lightly halfway up the eye. Place the color you choose over it near the lashes. If skin is reddish, use light brown shadow on bone.

The eyes should be made up more heavily for evening wear. Use a glistening film of gold over the bony part of the eyelid. Do not use gold or silver shadow in the daytime.

Mascara

Be sure the lashes are dry and the brush moist, but not too wet. Soak the brush a while in eye lotion. This makes the mascara thicker. Apply mascara thinly from roots to tips in upward strokes.

Coat each eyelash, and give an extra coat to the lashes at the outside corner of the eye.

If you have trouble with the lashes "fluttering" during application, try gently holding eyelid near the temple with your fingers, or try opening the mouth in a wide O to tense the muscles.

Use mascara on upper lashes only. If lower lashes are to be done, this must be just a faint touch of the brush.

Try tipping a solid color with another color—as green, violet or blue tips of lashes against black, or green tips against brown.

Use dark blue, violet or green mascara for evening.

If mascara seems too thick after application—wash brush, shake dry and "comb" out lashes. Wash brush after each application.

Hot Oil Shampoo

This is usually used in cases of dandruff and where the hair is dry and brittle, especially after too much exposure to sunshine.

First, brush the hair and scalp.

Second, apply warm olive oil or castor oil to the scalp with cotton. The warmer the oil the better, but do not get it hot enough to burn the scalp. Before you apply the oil, you should apply heat to the scalp with hot towels wrung dry or by use of a therapeutic lamp.

Third, massage the oil into the scalp as thoroughly as possible with the fingertips, as in shampooing.

Fourth, shampoo your hair as usual.

The hot oil shampoo may be done as often as every other day in severe cases of dandruff or dryness, but usually once a week is enough.

Variation (for difficult cases)

After step three above: Wring a turkish towel in hot water and wrap around head. Use several hot towels. This forces the oil into the scalp and the hair roots. Do not shampoo for approximately thirty minutes. Dry hair by hand and before completely dry, apply ointment or pomade to scalp. This will serve to heal the scalp if inclined to sensitiveness from the treatment.

The Beauty Bath

Make the most of your daily bath. Think of it not only as "the pause that refreshes," but also as the pause that softens and perfumes. Bathing is not only a social necessity, it can be a great treat and luxury as well. Utilize your bath time for cleansing, replenishing body oils, and over-all scenting. Submerged in water, relax and let go. Ease tensions. Prepare yourself for the rest of the day and evening to come.

If the water in your area is "hard" water, you might try a milk bath preparation which not only acts as a water softener but also serves as a fragrant additive.

After gently towel drying yourself, try one of the new aerosol bath powders. The ease of application, the lack of waste, the convenience of form will make you feel fabulous all over!

Also, you can find any number of new body-lotion preparations which are not only fragrant, but contain moisturizing properties to help keep your skin soft and silky.

In preparation for the bath, it is possible today to select a fragrance which comes in multiple forms to suit various needs.

For instance, one can find a perfume blend which is made up in: oil for the bath; perfumed soap; after bath oil; bath powder; friction-lotion cologne; perfume spray and essence. By using these preparations, you can retain and maintain your own unique aura, and that is one of the secrets of "Playing the Beauty Game" for keeps!

Part III

Life Is a Mystery—Solve It!

> *The greatest discovery of my generation is that human beings can alter their lives by altering their attitudes of mind.*
>
> —WILLIAM JAMES

The History and Mystery of Scent

CHAPTER EIGHT

People have been "Playing the Beauty Game" for cen-
turies. For instance, since the days of our earliest recorded history, fragrance and scent have been used not
only for religious and ritual purposes, but for seductive
beauty reasons as well. Nowhere in literature will you
find any more extensive use of perfumes, oils, incense and
unguents than you do throughout the Old and New Tes-
taments. To understand both the power and the purpose
of perfume, it is interesting to begin back in the Garden
of Eden where, according to the written word, men and
women first came together and started what became the
perpetual battle of the sexes.

In the pre-Christian era we find recorded evidence of
an extensive use of fragrances in the civilizations of
ancient Egypt, Greece and Rome. Looking toward the
continent of Asia, historical references tell us that scent
was used there hundreds of years before the birth of
Christ. Obviously, it is quite safe to state that ever since

47

Man was, he has used some form of scent as an important adjunct to his way of life.

Cleopatra has come down to us as the most famous female seductress through her use of perfumes, but the "habit" was also part of Biblical legend. Judith, when called upon to serve her people by seducing the general of an opposing army, prepared well for her task. As it says in the Bible, "She anointed herself with precious ointment, and decked herself bravely, to allure the eyes of all men that should see her."

Perfume always has been associated with pleasure and revelry. One young Roman ruler, addicted to banquets, wine, flowers and perfume, inaugurated various "fragrant" summer carnivals, each with a different color as its theme. There was a green festival, a pink festival, a violet festival, a blue festival, a special color for each warm summer's day. He blended wine with the most exotic additives, enhancing the bouquet of rose wine, for instance, by mixing it with fragrant fir-cone essence. He showered his banqueting halls with roses, lilies, violets, hyacinths and narcissi, and waded happily through oceans of blossoms. Having installed a reversible ceiling in his dining room, he tipped such quantities of violets and other flowers onto his guests that several of them lost their lives when they were unable to struggle out of the suffocating avalanche of blossoms and into open air! As an "extra added attraction," he would swim in his pool only if the water had been perfumed. Naturally, the rarest and most precious oils were provided whenever he went bathing with his court.

In the ancient city of Rome, the cult of perfumes, especially in connection with the rose, was carried to an extravagant degree and apparantly became a craze. When dining, wealthy nobles delighted in having elaborate fountains of constantly showering rose-water. Rose leaves were scattered on the floors of nobles' apartments and showered upon the heads of the guests from above. Rose garlands were placed on noble brows and festooned over their robes.

Perfumes were considered of such great value, that one Roman proverb advised noblemen never to leave their fine perfumes to their heirs! Instead, they were admonished to use all of their floral oils on themselves and will their heirs money. In other words, the use of fragrance was valued above all else, even gold.

In ancient Greece, particularly in Athens, the shops of perfumers became popular meeting places for the most fashionable members of society. You might say they were like our coffee houses where friends meet to gossip, to exchange confidences, to pass the time of day. The Greeks also were very fond of fragrant flowers. Ardent lovers would decorate the doors of their mistresses' homes in addition to bringing them armloads of beautiful blossoms.

In those times, healing properties were attributed to perfume, which may account for their great popularity. Rose water, used for medicinal purposes then, is a good example of a fragrant lotion which has lasted down through modern times.

The Greeks also carried on the Egyptian custom of placing flowers on the graves and tombs of the dead. Perfumes also played an important part in funeral ceremonies, and incense was thrown when the bodies of the dead were consumed by fire. The custom of offering flowers to the dead, which still survives, appears to have been world-wide from a time of great antiquity, and is thought to have arisen in the belief that since flowers and their odors were pleasing to man, their fragrance would be acceptable to the deities.

The first Queen Elizabeth's fondness for perfumes is

a matter of record. Her favorite special perfume was made as follows:

> Take 8 grains of musk and put in rose water 8 spoonfuls, 3 spoonfuls of damash water, and ¼ oz. of sugar. Boil for 5 hours and strain it.

At one point in early British history the use of perfumes was so excessive as to be regarded quite seriously. In fact, in 1770, a Bill was introduced into Parliament which read as follows:

> "That all women, of whatever rank, profession or degree, whether virgins, maids or widows, that shall from and after such Act, impose upon, seduce and betray into matrimony, any of his Majesty's subjects by the scents, paints, cosmetic washes, artificial teeth, false hair, Spanish wool (a wool impregnated with carmine used to colour the skin), iron stays, hoops, high-heeled shoes, and bolstered hips, shall incur the penalty of law now in force against witchcraft and like misdemeanours, and that, the marriage upon conviction shall be null and void."

The use of perfume in connection with gloves, especially in Napoleon's time, was so extensive that a variety of formulas for glove perfume has come down to us. Keep in mind that gloves were as essential to the dress of that day as any other garment worn. Much time, effort and great fortunes were employed in finding a glove scent of such allure that it tended to almost hypnotize those who came in contact with it. Two of the formulas are given below. The first is famous as a glove perfume, the second, a formula for making a perfume necklace.

Glove perfume: "Roses 1 lb., Orris 1 lb., Benzoin ½ oz., Storax ½ oz., Calamus 6 ozs., Essence of Citron 3 ozs., Coriander ½ oz., Girofle 6 ozs., lavender ¼ oz., Powder of Orange ½ oz., Rose wood 4 ozs., Santal ½ oz., Demy Muscade."

Perfume Necklace: "1 oz. of Benjamin, 1 oz. of Storax, 1 oz. of Labdanum. Heat in a mortar very hot, and beat all these gums to a perfect paste; in beating of it, put in 6 grains of Musk, 4 grains of Civet. When you have beaten all this to a fine paste, with your hands with rose water, roll it round betwixt your hands, and make holes in the beads, and so string them while they be hot."

By the early 17th Century, snuff taking was popular with both sexes, and citizens of style felt undressed without their snuff boxes. Presumably, snuff was used for medicinal purposes. For instance, by sniffing snuff, one had a tendency to sneeze, thereby clearing nasal passages, which in turn was supposed to alleviate headaches, soothe nerves and give one a restful night's sleep thereby resulting in a clearer head the following morning.

Whatever its purpose, snuff also was popular for its scent. Snuff, that quaint, old-fashioned sounding word, is actually nothing more than *perfumed* tobacco! As its use became more and more popular, many varieties were created, all employing the basic tobacco leaf, but adding to it various scents.

In France, snuff was perfumed with oil of cedar, jasmine, neroli, and dashes of musk and civit were added. When the very precious substance known as ambergris was mixed in, a special blend was made which was called the "Roman Odor."

Here are still more ideas taken from extensive records on the history and mystery of scent.

Ages ago, cinnamon was the basis for many love potions. Its aroma was supposed to be a powerful love charm.

It was once believed that the lily of the valley was a good heart tonic. Pansies were used in ancient times not only to make wine but also as an antiseptic.

Juniper berries were used by herbalists as a diuretic, as well as a basis for gin. Junipers were also believed to cure skin diseases. Oil of rosemary was a very popular remedy for headaches and was also used as a nerve tonic.

Spearmint leaves, when ground up and sprinkled on the head, were once believed capable of making people think better. Cinnamon oil was used in the treatment of flu and severe colds. Palm leaves were used to bind up and heal broken limbs.

In ancient Arabia, hosts sprinkled their guests with rose water not only as a token of friendship, but to ward off evil spirits. Mistletoe once was used for epilepsy and serious nerve disorders before it became a Christmas ornament.

Sweet basil, a plant which was regarded as sacred in ancient civilization, was used as a good luck omen. Many a Hindu slept with a leaf of basil stuck on his chest.

In "Playing the Beauty Game" today, you can forget about sleeping with basil leaves, but remember a dot of perfume on your pillow and bed linens can make playing the game much more exciting!

We have included this bit on the history and mystery of scent to emphasize the fact that today's beauty can and should take a leaf from the book of history. Let's face it; why should the ancient Greeks, Romans and Chinese be wiser and more alluring than the citizens of the 20th Century? The answer is simple—THEY SHOULDN'T!

Mood-Matched Scents

In addition to shopping for a fragrance which enhances YOUR unique self, remember you will undoubtedly wish to vary your selection of scents to fit both your mood as well as the occasion.

The following is a basic guide . . .

Young—Sweetly Flirtatious Mood

Choose floral scents and those giving off citrus fruit and/or grassy odors.

Sexy Mood

Choose a fragrance with a musk or civet base.

Sentimental-Nostalgic Mood

Perfumes with a jasmine, rose, or muguet (lily of the valley) scent fit this mood.

Wistfully Feminine

Scents with predominate notes of violet, heather, lilies, mimosa and cypress are perfect for this mood.

Very Romantic

Select scents blended of floral bouquets of Spring moss, or pick a fresh woody scent created for the young at heart.

Mysterious Mood

Choose scents of dominant Oriental spices and precious woods resembling an exotic Persian garden in full bloom.

Carefree Abandon

For this mood, pick a perfume composed of a wildflower bouquet, touched with roses and carnations and made with a musk base.

Perfume Groups

Florals are created from the true oils of natural flower blossoms such as Jasmine, Rose, Lilac, Violet. These rich natural oils are livened by the use and elaboration of a dozen ingredients to make the ideal portrait of a single flower. Almost all of them contain one or more of the precious three, *Oil of Roses,* for depth and richness; *Oil of Jasmine,* for vibrant liveliness;

Oil of Oranges, for airy and delicate grace. The fresh flower fragrance can be lightened and made lively with oil of tangerine, lime, lemon or bitter oranges.

Woodsy, Mossy, Leafy scents are created from green leaf and stem, bark and roots from the forest! These perfumes are fragrantly fortified with scented resins and sweet balsams extracted from the bark of trees. Most are built on a base of precious wood oils such as Sandalwood, Cedarwood, Bois de Rose (rosewood).

Orientals are generally composed of pungent, spicy and woodsy materials, such as tuberose, sandalwood, patchouli, vetiver, ilang-ilang, amber, balsam and musk. They usually outlast the more delicate floral scents. These odors are usually lightened and brightened with scents of flowers or a sharp note of citrus oil. These release the heavier basic scents. All is then bound together with the precious animal fixatives, musk, civet, or ambergris.

The Many Forms of Fragrance

Perfume	Scented drawer liner
Perfume oil	Perfumed soap flakes
Cologne (Spray Mist)	Perfumed nail polish
Body lotion	Flower-scented deodorant cologne
Sachet (dry)	Scented hair spray
Sachet (creme)	After bath lotion
Talc	Body oil
Dusting powder	Perfumed soap
Bath oil	After bath oil spray
Bubble bath	Pomander balls
Bath salts	Perfumed candles
Foaming bath oil	Incense
Floral scented bath drops	Scented facial tissues
Scented stationery	Snuff

NOTE: Keep this as a personal check list when you are planning to purchase items to enhance your TOTAL AURA.

How's Your Aura?

CHAPTER NINE

AURA: *". . . A subtle invisible essence said to emanate from a human body and to surround it like an atmosphere . . ."*

True feminine beauty is based on TOTAL impact. It is not limited to spectacular physical dimensions, nor to a classic profile—but rather exists in totality. As they say in today's advertising jargon, beauty should be "a package deal."

True feminine beauty is an aura . . . an emanation which the frankly *female* female exudes. True feminine beauty is a mystery, a mystique, a mathematically indefinable mixture of desire and reticence, temptation and temperance.

True feminine beauty is a well-modulated voice, an infectious laugh, enough knowledge to participate, to be aware, combined with the wisdom to listen and to care.

True feminine beauty is good grooming, good manners, good taste, a radiant personality. The beautiful woman is one who can conquer *all the male senses si-*

55

multaneously. In short, true feminine beauty is represented by a woman who is unique, who is unforgettable.

One of the most important and helpful ways to achieve "unforgettableness" is to surround yourself with a special scent. Acquire a fragrance trade-mark which sets you apart—not because it is so overpowering as to make men swoon at first sniff—but rather because it is subtle enough to keep a man enchanted, desiring, completely captive!

Just as "all that glitters is not gold," so, too, all that smells is not sweet. On these pages you will learn how to feel more beautiful through the specific use of fragrance. "Playing the Beauty Game" can be a snap once you've reached your top aura level!

We can show you how to intensify your individual aura through the application of some very basic sensual beauty secrets. This has nothing to do with physical beauty, or expensive clothes, or where you live, or how you earn your living. Your aura can be sensational, seductive, sweet, memorable, unforgettable—no matter who you are—provided you allow your imagination to take flight. Accept those suggestions which you find personally meaningful and use them as a guide to enhancing your total aura. By doing so, you will have gained knowledge of a great beauty technique.

In other sections of this book we have laid stress on the physical you; on your diet; on your exercise; on the subject of beauty surgery. Now a NEW dimension is added: one that affords you more clues on how to "Play the Beauty Game" advantageously by successfully surrounding yourself with scent.

Take from these pages what you will. *Remember, these words are not effective until and unless you per-*

sonally put them into practice. But once you *do* improve your fragrance potential, through the judicious use of perfumes and scents, your overall potential as a truly feminine female is greatly enhanced.

Getting down to specifics, what kind of an image do you *currently* project? Be honest with yourself! Now, what kind of an image would you wish to project if you had a choice? And you do! How do you want other people to see you? As a sex symbol? As the All-American girl? The cool debutante? The warmly passionate motherly type? The sophisticated career woman? The contented, loving housewife? A female on the prowl? Once you know what you are, who you are, and what you wish the world to see you as, then the clever use of perfumes comes into play. *Perfumes. Plural.*

Why limit yourself to only one image? *The wise female is many women.* She changes her image to fit the mood, the season, the occasion, the company. A woman may project the All-American ski bunny image in winter, the well organized, introspective young matron in the fall, a provocative bikini clad beauty in the summer, and a smoldering sex pot when those leaves of autumn start to turn. For a woman to reflect all of these images in one body, she requires knowledge, skill, planning—*and a bit of help.*

Fashion contributes to a woman's mood. An exciting invitation to a formal dinner party influences the style and image she should project. On the next day, if the same woman is invited to go riding, or to the beach, her image must change to fit the occasion.

Thus you see how grooming, make-up, wardrobe all help to create the desired illusion. And along with these surface trappings comes the necessity for a wise choice of perfumes, colognes, hand lotions, bath oils, etc. *Every woman has the need for that which cannot be seen but which is always present—a uniquely fragrant image.*

While the statistical influence of scent on the sex life of primitive peoples cannot be measured precisely, we *do* have evidence that smell has had a marked influence on relationships between people since man evolved.

Nose rubbing as a sign of affection is a ritual based on closeness, the actual "sniffing" of others. You all know much has been written about the Eskimo custom of nose rubbing used much in the same way as we use the kiss.

Dancing, embracing, all forms of close human contact call into play not only visual sensations but olfactory ones as well.

Perfume—when suited to the individual—should ideally give off a subtle scent which has the potential of arousing or inducing a romantic association. Face it, that's what the "Beauty Game" is all about—isn't it?

This is a good time to state another thought: *the same scent does not suit every woman.* There are scents which enhance specific hair color and complexion types. There are even *finer* distinctions, including the fact that *different* fragrances may be used by the *same* woman to coincide with a variety of moods. The most important factor, once you have selected perfumes to suit your individual personality and mood, is to make the most effective use of these fragrances.

The truly feminine woman uses fragrance to enhance her charms every hour of the day, in every room of her house, on various parts of her body, and as a traveling companion wherever she goes. Only by a knowledge of and a total use of the correct fragrances is the modern female utilizing one of the most provocative weapons at her command. Some of these suggestions may seem far out, but don't knock them until you've at least tried them. After all, never before has a woman had the opportunity to utilize so much fragrance with so little trouble.

Choosing the proper scents becomes a matter of experimentation. All little girls, at sometime or other, are given gifts of sweetly perfumed soaps, bubble bath, and various other toilet articles. A young girl's first identification with scent is through gifts given to her before she is old enough for personal discrimination. When a girl reaches her teens, she may have a tendency to go overboard when she first realizes that scents are meant for more than just pleasing the wearer. Frequently a girl will adopt the fragrances which her mother or other female members of the family use. Mainly this is for economic reasons and again not out of any personal preference. However, when a girl reaches the age where she makes her *own* purchase of a scent, her "fragrance education" must begin.

Millions and millions of dollars are spent each year by leading perfumers and cosmetic makers all with one specific purpose: to get you to buy their product. At first, it is easy to be influenced into buying a certain perfume because of the fabulous advertising campaign which goes with it. This breaks down in several ways, either through constant repetition of a brand name, or else because of a specific name of a scent which sounds alluring. The discriminating woman must learn *not* to be lured into buying any perfume either because of its heavy advertising campaign, or its brand name, *unless the specific product suits her own individual personality and enhances her charms.*

In recent years, certain well known perfumes have been widely purchased through the influence of famous women. Who can ever forget the charming quote attributed to the late Marilyn Monroe when she was questioned about posing for that now famous nude calendar. When asked if she had really posed without anything on, she smiled sweetly and said, "No, the radio was on . . . and I was *wearing* Chanel No. 5."

Not too much later, Elizabeth Taylor, upon being interviewed by a national magazine, mentioned her favorite perfume, an exotic gardenia blend. Overnight the sales of this fragrance sky-rocketed. In both cases, the actresses involved mentioned fragrances which suited *them* personally. Yet literally thousands of women rushed to buy these specific products merely because two famous sex symbols had mentioned them. While some of the women might well have been purchasing a scent which was indeed good for them, more than likely the majority were not! We are trying to say that advertising per se is not bad or harmful. Still, you must let your own brain and nose be your guide in selecting the proper perfume for your own special aura.

To really "Play the Beauty Game" to the fullest extent, it would be marvelous if you could design an ideal setting to enhance your own unique and total aura. If you could, it would begin on the path leading to your front door. There would be a profusion of rose bushes and other scented flowers lining the walk. Crossing over the threshold into your entranceway, one would get the next awareness of YOU. If it were dinnertime, there would be a generous sniff of aromatic dishes cooking in another part of the house. These odors would not be indelicate or overpowering, but merely present in the air, subtle, tantalizing, giving a hint of the delicious meal to come.

Your living room would be tastefully furnished, employing colors and textures of fabrics especially selected to enhance YOU. There would be subtle tones, plus touches of vibrant colors, fireplace logs burning bright orange, and a vase or two of freshly cut flowers. You would have prepared your living room in another way by anointing several electric bulbs in your lamps with drops of your favorite perfume. As each bulb was lit and became warm, it would bathe the room not only in a soft glow of light, but also it would give off gentle hints of your own personal scent. While your family and/or special guests were pouring cocktails from a freshly mixed batch, prepared in advance, you would be in the bedroom putting on the final touches.

Earlier, you would have relaxed in a tub scented with bath oil. You would have emerged, dried off, and powdered yourself with talc or dusting powder. You would have gone into your bedroom, opened your dresser drawer, and taken out your finest lingerie, which was already delicately scented by perfumed paper with which you had lined your drawers.

After putting on your inner-garments, and before stepping into your dress, or hostess pajamas, you would have applied several sprays of a good deodorant and anti-perspirant to insure an evening of freshness. Then you would have taken a small square of cotton, saturated it with enough drops of your special perfume to make the pad moist, and then tucked it into the folds of your breast, fastened by your bra. There the cotton would remain all evening giving an extra note of fragrance as it was continually warmed by the heat of your own body. Before dressing, you would apply your favorite scent to those important places on your body which guarantee the most lasting fragrance: inside each wrist; behind each knee; behind each ear; a few drops dabbed on various parts of your hair. Then you would have dressed and, with a final touch, you would have sprayed your favorite scent upon your neck and shoulders.

As you entered the living room, you would present a total picture of both fragrant and visual loveliness. As you walked into your living room, you would be complimented by everything surrounding you. While your guests were pouring you a cocktail, you would make a final check of your dining room table. You would light a pair of tapering candles (scented, of course). As a centerpiece, you would have a bowl of freshly cut flowers, giving off a fragrance planned to compliment your own special perfume scent. Once you had double-checked the table, and taken a peek into the kitchen to see that everything was under control, you would rejoin your guests, spend a few quiet moments sipping your cocktail, and then announce that dinner is ready.

While your company sat in amazement, you would bring to the table a variety of dishes overflowing with delectable scents and looking very appetizing. Your salad bowl would be cool and crisp. Your vegetables would be gently seasoned. Your main course, be it meat, fish, or fowl, would be enhanced by the use of aromatic spices. On the table a bottle of wine would sit waiting to be poured. Throughout the meal your companions could not help admiring the total picture of yourself which you have presented. When the main course was almost completed, you would set a pot of coffee nearby until its rhythmic perking and special aroma came drifting into the dining room. You might end with a simple dessert and an elegant snifter of brandy. Whatever you served, it would be done beautifully, tastefully, fragrantly.

The balance of the evening would depend upon your guests and your specific plans. But whatever came, it would be carried off in the same truly feminine manner. At the end of the evening, your guests would walk back down the same path they had entered a short while before, taking with them the sensation of *your* aura, *your* presence—that *total you* which had enchanted them while you were together and which will linger with them while you are apart.

This ideal evening spent "Playing the Beauty Game" is very important whether designed to share with company, or for spending with the man you love. Either way, it will be fun—and you will leave a lasting impression of beauty.

Play the Beauty Game: Psych and Scent Your Man!

CHAPTER TEN

Stop! Think! Scent!

What lovely female cannot be even lovelier with the wise use of a "girl's best friend," fragrance?

Scent should not be limited to those "going-out-dressing-up" occasions. After all, it is much more important to be exciting and alluring for the man in your lift than for the neighborhood bridge club.

Stop! Think! Scent!

In preparing to retire, dot a bit of your favorite fragrance on your shoulders . . . at the nape of the neck . . . behind each ear . . . over the heartbeat . . . at the pulse points inside each wrist . . . another few drops on your pillow. Now you and your man are ready to float off to dreamland happily "intoxicated" by the aura which surrounds you both!

You say you have no special man? Well, all the more reason to make yourself SCENTSATIONAL. While we do not profess to be guides to the lovelorn, we have proof positive that the clever use of fragrance *has* helped snag more sweethearts than you can possibly imagine.

How? Well, assuming you have picked out a potential mate, choose a fragrance which will reach out and tug at his heartstrings. How? The answers are many and varied, as varied as the types of men a woman is apt to encounter. Therefore, while this chapter cannot encompass a basic handbook of every conceivable type, there ARE certain broad categories of males, and certain general rules which, if followed, can be extremely helpful.

1. MR. OUTDOORS: Is your P.M. (Potential Mate) the athletic type? If so, in what way? Does he *actively* participate, or is he merely a rabid spectator? The distinction between Mr. Outdoors, who plays to win, and Mr. Sports Enthusiast, who likes to watch others win, is obvious. With the active Mr. Outdoors, we will assume that to have made the initial contact you, too, have a well-coordinated body and a natural talent for handling a tennis racket, or swimming the breast stroke, or skiing when snow is on the ground. If this is so, you are undoubtedly the clean-cut, all-American type who usually chooses a very sweet, subtle scent. If you have followed this general pattern up to now, *go one step further.* Use your sweet, subtle fragrance during the daytime, or for those evenings when you actively engage in sports. *But be prepared to pull a switch.*

Once you know he's Mr. Right, and you have a feeling that he thinks of you as Miss Right, it is time to select the most *potent* ammunition purchasable. Pick the time he asks you out to dinner (when you know it will be a dressup occasion) to treat yourself to a scent-type you have never used before. Leave your bottle of sweet floral scent unopened. Select a sexy, richly warm body perfume in the jasmine or muguet range. Buy this scent in several *different* forms. Try a bath oil, a dusting powder, and a perfume or cologne all in the same line. Arrange your schedule so you have enough time for a beauty bath. Let your new scent saturate your skin and surround you with a whole new image.

Before you dress, sprinkle some of your new scent on a cotton pad. Tuck it into your bra so the fragrance will continue to surround you throughout the evening. While we offer no written guarantee that a switch in scent will automatically bring you a proposal, don't be a bit surprised if Mr. Outdoors succumbs. Why? Well, assuming he is already attracted to you for your companionship at outdoor events, your subtle switch to a slyly seductive scent is likely to set his mind spinning in other directions, such as toward activites of a more *indoor* variety. Try it and see. Have fun! Good luck!

On the other hand, if the Mr. Outdoors you know is strictly the spectator type, it stands to reason you are the same breed of cat. Assuming this is so, that you attend sports events either out of genuine interest, or because your female instinct tells you this is the thing to do, then you are most probably the type of woman who tends toward sophistication in both dress and scent. Therefore, YOUR SWITCH IS IN THE OPPO-SITE DIRECTION. Assuming your ordinarily wear a sexy, heavily alluring fragrance, go out and buy a new perfume which also suits you, but which is of an entirely *different* type. CHOOSE A SCENT THAT IS SOMEWHAT LITTLE GIRLISH. Perhaps something in the sweet pea or lilac family.

Once you have chosen your "little girl" scent, select an informal occasion—preferably a night when he is coming to dinner. It goes without saying that you should outdo yourself in the kitchen department. But follow through in the *fragrance* department as well. Select a charming, informal *un*-seductive dress to wear. Take a beauty bath and surround yourself with your new girlish aura. By the law of averages, *this* should do the trick. He already knows you can be a woman of the world, now you will have shown him you can also be the girl of his heart and his hearth. Try it. You have nothing to lose but your last name! You see, "Playing the Beauty Game" can be fun!

2. MR. BUSY EXECUTIVE: Moving on to another type of male, let us assume that your Potential Mate is very much a Mr. B.E. (Busy Exec). Of necessity, he would be a no-nonsense type, the efficient, take-charge male who likes to run the show. In order to appeal to this type, you are undoubtedly Miss Efficiency, too. You already have learned that your dates will run on a tight schedule, and that when Mr. B.E. says he will pick you up at seven, he expects you to be ready at seven. If you've been dating him for any length of time, you already have proven your ability to fit into his very ordered life. But now, PULL THE SWITCH. Show him the other side of your nature. You see, down deep, even a B.E. needs to unwind and become Mr. E.G. every now and then. E.G., of course, stands for EASY-GOING.

So here is your plan: At the first opportunity, preferably on a night when he expects to come to your home for a well-planned meal, cooked just to his taste, and served exactly on schedule, have a big surprise waiting for him. Be completely unpredictable! *Don't be all dressed and ready when he arrives.* Let him sit in the living room by himself for a few moments. Let him relax, unwind, and take notice of his surroundings.

Let him drink in the atmosphere, the sumptuous scents of a dinner still cooking. Most of all, let him begin to wonder where you are and what you are up to.

Where you are is in your bedroom. *What you are up to is shifting your external image by altering your usual aura.* You will have prepared in advance for this evening by having purchased some wistfully feminine scent, a fragrance reminiscent of the old South, when magnolias were in bloom and mint julips, rather than martinis, were the order of the day. You will be putting on extremely feminine lounging pajamas. But first you will be adding the final touches of a mimosa-scented fragrance guaranteed to make you as much of a *femme fatale* as Scarlett O'Hara. When you finally make your entrance, Mr. B.E. will be curiously bug-eyed. You will have momentarily caught him off-guard. For the first time, he will be uncertain as to what is coming next. This is a method of "Playing the Beauty Game" to the hilt. I leave the rest to your imagination. Just think to yourself: What would Scarlett O'Hara have done? Then go to it!

3. MR. PROFESSIONAL MAN: If you already have been dating a P.M. for a while, then you know he is one of the hardest types to pin down on a *permanent* basis. If your doctor, lawyer or professor hasn't been married during his years of schooling and early training, then you have a problem. A woman seeking the affection of this type of man enters into the relationship knowing that more than likely the man she's trying to land already has a Mistress, a Mistress who will be his first love no matter what. Her name is Medicine, or Law, or Education. She is the most powerful rival a flesh and blood woman has to contend with. But it *can* be done—if you "Play the Beauty Game" wisely.

If your P.M. is a doctor, you're in *big* trouble to

start with. Assuming a man has gone through medical school, internship, residency, and is now in practice, there is nothing about a woman he doesn't know, hasn't seen, can't automatically diagnose. Therefore, the *usual* feminine tricks won't work. The "average" doctor is not subject to the ordinary temptations which other men fall for. He has seen all the bodies, touched all the skin, become familiar with the female anatomy to such an extent that he is quite blasé and un-reachable in the *normally* "seductive ways." So how do you set about winning the heart of a man who can tell you how many valves and chambers yours has? Simple! Analyze him. He's bound to have an Achilles' Heel. For almost his entire adult life, he has gone by the books, the charts, followed the prescribed ways for dealing with people. *He needs to be surprised on the most basic level.* You see, the truth is that in many ways a doctor's life is quite narrow—especially when it comes to the social sphere. The normally dedicated medical man does not have time for much tomfoolery. Therefore, while he cannot be "gotten to" on some levels, he can be an absolute push-over on others. (Colleagues, forgive me!)

If you are dating a doctor, you already are neat and orderly. Usually medical men abhor chaos and mess. Untidy apartments, dirty kitchens, a frumpy looking woman, are things he usually runs away from. Now, assuming you are the type who appeals to the antiseptic doctor, the next step is very fundamental. Buy the most *demurely* sophisticated dress you can find. Let it be a high neck, long-sleeved, terribly basic gown. Wear a simple strand of pearls. Select a scent about as far away from those he is used to as possible. *Try a fragrance which suggests carefree abandon.* Select a perfume in the wild flower bouquet range, highlighted by either a hint of roses, or carnations, and underscored by a trace of musk. This fragrance, plus a seemingly simple, basic dress can be startling to him. In contrast to clinical white, you will appear in alluring black. In contrast to antiseptic smells, you will be scented by fragrance that reminds him of those by-gone days before the world of X-rays and needles became his way of life. *He will recognize in you an oasis:* a safe, sweet, serene island far removed from the strain of his normal days. If this doesn't do the trick, forget it. He'll probably wind up marrying a nurse!

The second category of P.M. is Mr. L.E. (Legal Eagle). He is the gentleman who spends his life involved in other peoples' lives. Usually he is a little less rigid and narrow in social scope than the doctor. Depending of course on the kind of law he practices, there are numerous variations on this theme. However, remember one thing—just as the doctor knows what women are like biologically, inside and out, so the lawyer knows most women *intellectually* and *emotionally*. There are very few tricks or feminine wiles that an attorney will fall for. During the course of his study and training, he has heard every story that the human mind can invent. If he handles many matrimonial cases, he also has seen some women who aren't very pretty. He's heard intimate details of married life which are enough to scare any man away from falling into the same trap. To win the love of a lawyer, a woman needs to be Portia-like herself. Either that, or else so incredibly naive that she represents the opposite of all her Mr. L.E. comes into contact with. Most lawyers can be appealed to on the homey, nostalgic level of life they knew before they entered the world of writs, torts and *habeus corpus*. Therefore, whatever scent you normally wear, try switching to an Old-World fragrance represented by muguet (lily of the valley) or jasmine. If you already are using this type of scent, expand upon it. Add a touch of mystery to your mood. Try a fragrance whose dominant notes are Oriental in nature. A scent which resembles an exotic Persian garden in full bloom is the best! If that doesn't do the trick, cross the barrister off your list and look for a less complicated subject. Meanwhile, you'll still have fun "Playing the Beauty Game."

The third category of Professional Man we have labeled "Mr. Professor". The rules that apply to this type also go well with the scientist, the dedicated engineer, or any cerebral type who lives in an ivory tower, and whose Mistress is research, knowledge, progress and very often *the unknown*. The man whose daily life is spent in the proverbial Halls of Ivy, or in a lab, or in a library, needs a *complete change* when it comes to the woman in his life. He needs a *non-technical type*. A lovely lady whose intelligence is there when necessary, and tucked beneath soft chiffon and lace at other times. The way to this man's heart is on the most romantic level. Select a fragrance blended of floral bouquets, of spring moss, or a fresh woody scent which represents the perpetually young at heart. For this man, who has dedicated his life to knowledge, is still in many ways a boy at heart. He is a man of perpetual youth. The very nature of his occupation revolves around interest in future generations. For a grown man to be interested in tomorrow, he must retain much of the idealistic-little-boy quality. *That* kind of man most readily succumbs to the *ultimate* in romantic imagery.

4. MR. MUSCLES: Unlike our Mr. Outdoors man, this type is *not* the athletic participant or spectator. He is the man you see on those TV commercials with a

tattoo, a man who would really rather "fight than switch." His occupation involves great physical strength and dexterity. He is a mechanic, a hard-working craftsman, someone who uses his brawn more than, or at least as much as, his brain. Usually this type is so overwhelmingly masculine in appearance that he looks as though he has the strength of a granite mountain. Well, maybe he does when it comes to his work, but usually he is as softhearted inside as a mound of sand. This rough and ready male adores his opposite, the soft, cuddly female. With rare exception, Mr. Muscles doesn't like a girl who can handle a monkeywrench or fix a leaky faucet. That is *his* area. He does not want his woman messing around under any sinks. To win Mr. Muscles, you must be the youthfully flirtatious type, even if you have said goodbye to your twenty-first birthday more years ago than you care to remember. *To be young in the way we use the term has nothing to do with the years of a calendar.* It involves the *inner* spirit as reflected by the *outer* appearance and behavior.

Select fragrances with a floral base which are highlighted by citrus fruits or grassy odors. Dress in the most feminine clothes you can find. Leave the tailored slacks and blouses to the other women. Find yourself a pretty, bright, utterly feminine dress that reflects your own young-at-heart spirit. If you do this, Mr. Muscles will turn into a plate of jelly just long enough to ask that all important question. He will, if he reacts "normally", that is! If he doesn't, forget him and "Play the Beauty Game" with someone else.

5. MR. CONSERVATIVE: We have nicknamed this type "Mr. Homebody". His conservative nature is reflected not only in his occupation but in his social life as well. This male can be found in many fields of endeavor. *With him it is not so much what he does for a*

living, but rather his general attitude toward life. He is the opposite of the flamboyant extrovert. He is the quiet steady type. A reliable man who finds his niche, fills it, and stays with it, not because he's in a rut, but because he is doing what he wants to, period. This man usually cannot be nagged, prodded, or changed. He shuns loud parties. He runs from the "mad whirl" toward serenity.

Because of his nature, Mr. Conservative is easy to spot *but hard to figure out.* Usually this type appears to be somewhat unemotional. A woman often finds it difficult to approach him. In his own way, like the Professional Man, the normal female tricks will *not* work on him, and in fact are quite repugnant to his inner nature. *Subtlety is the key.* If you are dating Mr. Conservative, you must toss aside any heavily spiced fragrances. Pick something subtle which suits you and also appeals to Mr. C. Remember, he is not the type who can be hit over the head and overpowered by an overly aggressive female. *You must steal Mr. Conservative's heart*—when he *isn't looking.*

The first scent we'd suggest does *not* come from the perfume counter, but from your local market. This is the type of man who must be wooed *simultaneously* on several levels: through the kitchen as well as through your own personal wiles. So try baking something with a homespun flavor—such as gingerbread. Plan an evening for him which will begin the moment he walks through the door and gets his first whiff of your cooking. Gingerbread might well be preceded by a hearty aromatic meal (see recipes in the "Spice Up Your Life" section). While your main dish is simmering on the stove, you will be simmering in a beauty bath totally surrounded by a fragrance his dear old mother might have used. Lavender is our top suggestion for this occasion. Lavender with its subtle aroma makes a man think of Mama and home and respectability. If your Mr. Conservative spends an evening dining on a hearty home-cooked meal, and sniffing gingerbread, all the while surrounded by you and your lavender lilt, and he still doesn't succumb, then forget him and look elsewhere. Any man who could resist this "ploy" is almost bound to be a confirmed bachelor of the hard-core variety.

You have read about five basic types of men and the unique suggestions for ways to reach them on a permanent basis. If your Prospective Mate does not fit into any one of these categories, at least study the suggested guidelines and apply the general rules to your own potential Mr. Right.

In analyzing a man, always remember to take into consideration his profession, his background, the things and people he ordinarily comes into contact with. Be sure you know his pattern and how to fit into it nicely. Of course, every feminine ploy is a gamble. But then, as we said before, *all of life is a game of chance.* Who can say that this method of "Psyching and Scenting" your man is not every bit as reliable as the mechanical computer which so many women are turning to these days? So before you ask a metal robot to make you a match, try your own female instincts and natural feminine talents. You can always resort to a machine—if necessary! Just keep in mind that "Playing the Beauty Game" can be your most potent weapon—and you know what they say about all weapons being fair in love and war!

The Sweet Scent
of Success

1. *How perfume lasts:* Perfumes are made lasting by certain ingredients that hold the complex oils together. Perfume must have coverage, not just a spot touched to the skin. As precious oils are released into the air, they evaporate, but this same evaporation is what "breathes out" so deliciously. Naturally, light scents like colognes or mists are more fugitive than heavier, stronger essences, such as perfumes and pure oils, which are more lasting.

2. *How to apply perfume:* Perfume must be used lavishly by the standards of American women (used to applying it sparingly), and renewed often during the day and evening. Certain spots on the body give out more warmth and therefore are best conductors for fragrance. The wrists . . . the crook of the elbow . . . behind the ears . . . the crook of the knees . . . at the temples. Just as lipstick or powder is renewed during the day, so

75

perfume should be renewed again and again. Remember to carry a purse atomizer.

3. *How to keep perfume:* Keep the bottles in their original boxes in a cool spot. This keeps light from fading the color. Keep tightly corked against evaporation and *use* the perfume instead of hoarding it. Unlike wines, perfume does not need aging. It is a perfect product when bottled.

A fine, perfectly balanced scent has great lasting powers. The very nature of the flower oils and fixatives lend themselves to diffusion, giving off their fragrance in the air; but the fragrance must be used lavishly if the scent is to retain its greatest intensity. Evaporation robs the strongest aroma of its highest pitch, so perfume should be renewed, and often, to keep its beauty constant.

Great perfumers suggest that perfume should be sprayed for the greatest aura of fragrance. Spray perfume on the body after the bath—the fine scented moisture settles on the skin and the warmth of your body renews the delightful aroma again and again.

Scent Tips

Tuck a saturated cotton pad in your purse or your bra.

Spray the hem of your skirt, your hankie, your hair, the inside crown of your hat.

Did you know that Napoleon scented his gloves with violet and the Empress Josephine scented the draperies of her boudoir with musk?

Sachet powder is wonderful used on the skin or scattered under the paper lining of bureau drawers. The old-fashioned idea of sachet bags placed among your lingerie, gloves and hankies is still a delightful one. Use perfume mist when you *make pin curls*. Shake some in the rinse water for your lingerie. And for refreshing sleep, spray your favorite scent on your pillow, or dot the lamp bulb beside your bed. Spray linen and clothes closets.

Remember, a "dab" of perfume behind the ear is not enough! Applying perfume as it should be used provides a woman with one of her greatest romantic weapons—the lingering aura that becomes intimately associated with her personality and charm.

Part IV

Life Is a Challenge—Meet It!

*It is never too late to be
what you might have been.*

—GEORGE ELIOT

The Good Life

Featuring the "Durable Dynamo Diet"

CHAPTER TWELVE

No one works at achieving lasting beauty harder than today's motion picture and television star. Let's face it —when the exterior appearance is vital to success, one moves heaven and earth to perfect it. When a healthy body is essential to one's craft, obtaining it and *maintaining* it is a must.

For many years, dozens of Hollywood's top stars have pursued the very special way of life which is found inside the doors of a place called "The Good Life."

Located in North Hollywood, California, a few blocks from Universal and Warner Brothers Studios, and a few minutes away from NBC and the Valley branch of CBS, this health food store has become a mecca for the "beauty seekers".

Daily, you can see your favorite celebrities as they leave the delicacies of a catered studio luncheon behind to eat a simple, nourishing, tasty meal at "The Good Life."

Owned and operated by Julie and Frank Mackey, "The Good Life" has become a complete way of life for many people. Frequently, the Mackeys are called

81

upon to suggest a star's nutritional plan of eating, a plan most often followed not only by the celebrity but by his or her entire family as well.

Don't get the wrong impression—"The Good Life" is *not* reserved only for V.I.P.'s. Everyone can partake of the type of life-style represented at a modern-day health food establishment. It is but typical of those stores which offer a variety of good sound nutritional products which can be beneficial to any who care to try them.

We owe the Mackeys a debt of gratitude for their help in formulating the DURABLE DYNAMO DIET especially for you!

The "Durable Dynamo Diet"

CHAPTER THIRTEEN

In order to be truly effective, a diet should embody a way of life which can be followed until the desired weight is lost—and then followed to maintain and stabilize the weight loss.

Fad diets come and go. However, a person who is overweight, with a tendency to bulk, needs to find and follow an eating plan which lasts more than a few days, or a couple of weeks. Proper eating must be *your* new way of life if you want to successfully "Play the Beauty Game."

While we do not say that the "Durable Dynamo Diet" is the *only* way, we can assure you that it *is* one way to health and beauty on a permanent basis.

However, to go a step further, you *will* find other diets in this book, even a few which are of the fad-phenomena type. We offer these, in addition to the "Durable Dynamo" and "T = T & T" diets so that you, as an individual, may select your own method for weight loss. The choice, milady, is yours!

The basic design of the "Durable Dynamo Diet," hereafter referred to as "DDD", reduced to simple arithmetic proportions, is:

to keep proteins above 160 grams daily
to keep saturated fats below 25 grams daily
to keep carbohydrates below 60 grams daily
to keep calories below 1500 calories daily

There are four essentials to the diet each of which has been formulated to work in conjunction with the other three. In order to take advantage of the amazing results you must follow this precept. Scientifically (excluding individual glandular cases), you cannot avoid losing weight on this diet.

To explain the advantage of this diet we must give you a simple key to the danger points inherent in other diets which are in wide usage. The average diet which only stresses low calories is invariably low in nutrients. This causes fatigue and flabby tissues. While the weight may come off, you are *not* helping your over-all physical appearance. With a diet based on the principle of high protein, you run into the problem of high calories. This does *not* help the body's cholesterol level, and also raises one very dangerous probability: If there is the slightest deviation, if you cheat even a little, more often than not weight loss will stop, reverse itself and you will gain weight!

On the diets which only stress low-saturated fatty foods, you run into the same drawbacks as you do with the average low calory diet. In other words, fatigue and flabby tissue are part and parcel of this regime, too.

Finally, among the diets most commonly in vogue

now, those stressing low carbohydrates, feature foods that are too high in saturated fats.

Only by combining, controlling and balancing the number of proteins, saturated fats, carbohydrates and calories which are consumed daily can you have a formula for weight reduction which is scientifically and mathematically workable.

There is one other factor which we should re-emphasize because it embodies interesting facts of which the average weight watcher rarely has been informed.

The serious failure of many so called high protein diets lies in quality. Before we can attempt to apply the words "high protein" to a reducing diet, we must first have some understanding of what high quality means in a protein.

Today, many people go on so-called high protein diets. They consult the charts and find that soy beans are high in protein, as is cottage cheese, or vegetables, or nut proteins of some sort. Therefore, they feel they are following a high protein diet.

However, because a high quality protein will burn in a perfect ratio—that is, one gram of a top quality protein will burn 3 grams of carbohydrate in the body—we must first understand what "high quality" means in regard to protein.

Many organizations publish a standard of what they call "Recommended Daily Dietary Allowances of Protein." To do this, they set an amount for protein intake that they believe will provide the needed essential amino acids and the total amino acids which include the non-essential ones. We believe the nutritionist of the future, who specializes in reducing problems, will not speak of protein but only of amino acids, of which the proteins are made.

Most nutritionists, even those of high standing, have

learned their amino acids by name and then forgotten them, perhaps a dozen times over. But the most practical approach to the problem is to consider only the *three* most important, because without these, the assimilation of all the others is in jeopardy. These three are: *methionine, phenylalanine* and *tryptophan* (meth-eye-o-neen, fen-a-lal-a-neen and trip-to-fane.)

For example, cereal proteins have a *low* biologic value because they contain *limiting* amounts of some essential amino acids. But proteins derived from animal sources are more likely to have a better pattern and quantity of these essentials and, therefore, a higher biologic value.

Most published charts hedge on their figures. For instance, they will set a figure desirable for a 154 lb. man at 65 grams of pure dietary protein per day, or a woman of 128 lbs. at 55 grams. But they qualify this by saying:

1. This protein is *assumed* to be of high quality
2. This protein is meant to include a well balanced diet.
3. This protein must include the recommended quantities of essential amino acids.
4. This protein should include substantial percentages of animal protein.

Therefore, these standards really are just a guessing game and offer no guarantee that the protein intake will be sufficient in the specified amount.

More than likely, we should double the standard recommendations. To do that, our hypothetical 154 lb. man would need to get about two pounds of porterhouse steak, or cottage cheese, or two dozen eggs, or four quarts of milk, just to mention a few foods. With all the concern today about cholesterol levels, you should recognize at once that our man would be getting too much saturated fat in his food with such a diet. That is why we believe in supplementing the diet with a high quality organ meat protein (available in powder or tablet form), one that is a mixture of liver, brain, kidney, heart, etc. This contains a fine balance of the quality amino acids we are talking about, namely *methionine, phenylalanine* and *tryptophan.*

Now what does this all mean to reducing? To understand why these high protein diets work (when they are properly used) we must first understand a few facts about the energy requirements of the body and how they are met. The body uses the following items in this order for energy:

1. Dietary and blood carbohydrates
2. Dietary fats
3. Body fat
4. Dietary protein
5. Body protein

Since the *energy requirements* of the body are met before all others, the higher quality protein formula will result in fast weight loss because body fat is used before protein food.

Major Recommendations for Protein Requirements in Reducing

1. The total protein intake should be almost double the generalized minimums, double or more.

2. The proteins used should generally be of the highest quality and best balance of the three most important amino acids, as well as being adequate in all the essential ones.

3. Proteins of high quality are an *absolute necessity* for a sound weight reduction program.

4. The foods which contain all three essential amino acids in good balance are all meat, fish, poultry, eggs and milk. The organ meats (liver, brain, kidney and heart) contain these essential amino acids in the *best* balance. Therefore, if your diet does not include organ meats, you should supplement it with a protein concentrate which contains the correct balance of *methionine, phenylalanine* and *tryptophan.*

5. ALWAYS be sure than enough *unsaturated* fatty acids (good vegetable oils) are included in the daily diet in order to help keep down the cholesterol level in the blood stream. This is particularly important on a high protein diet. By good oils we mean those that are polyunsaturated.

To sum up once again, a good quality protein burns in the proper ratio. One gram of a good protein will burn three grams of carbohydrate in the blood stream. This is a fact which has been proven in a laboratory. On the other hand. a "bad quality" protein, such as the soy bean, has a poor distribution of amino acids.

We are distressed by the voluminous books written for dieters which go into enormous amounts of clinical studies and medical data that cannot possibly be readily understood by the layman. It is not a question of intelligence, or rate of comprehension, but merely an excess of statistics which get in the way of the main objective, to safely lose weight, and to keep the weight off!

In our opinion, both the "Durable Dynamo Diet" and the one we call "T = T & T," are most realistic in their approach to scientific weight loss. If you chose to follow either of them, you will achieve results.

Once again, we advise you to consult your physician before undertaking any diet plan.

Now, go to it! Remember, life is a game of chance.

By "Playing the Beauty Game" with enthusiasm, plus the proper mental outlook, you can make every day of your life healthier and much more fun—forever.

Perhaps you are not aware of what happens to your body when you drastically change your way of eating. In layman's terms, it would be easiest to say that the body goes into a sort of shock condition, until, miraculously, it eventually adjusts to your new way of living.

Helping your body to adjust to a new diet means several key things. It means helping yourself to withstand temptations by inducing the most advantageous physical and mental state. It means giving your whole network of nerves an opportunity to realign itself until it reaches the point where it will not shoot off those miserable hunger pangs that lead many a dieter to the nearest hot fudge sundae!

What can be done to try and assure such a stable frame of mind and body? Well, over the years, we have found that by taking a formula of high B complex with C tablet two times a day, the average person is able to go on and stay on any diet for more prolonged periods than without vitamins.

You will find such tablets at your neighborhood drug or health food store. In general seek a tablet which will supply somewhat the following:

General Formula

B Complex with C

each tablet to contain in the range of:

Vitamin B1	10 - 25 mg.
Vitamin B2	10 - 30 mg.
Vitamin B6	10 - 25 mg.
Vitamin B12	25 - 75 mg.
Vitamin C	200 - 300 mg.

Niacinamide   25 - 50 mg.
Pantothenic Acid   50 - 100 mg.
In a base of Torumel Yeast

Naturally, as with all suggestions in this book, consult your own personal physician before you begin taking any tablets.

French Dressing

½ cup Safflower oil   1 tbs. Honey
¼ cup Sesame seed oil   2 tbs. Water
¼ cup Olive oil   1 clove Garlic
1 cup Wine vinegar

Salt, pepper and season to personal taste. Suggested herbs and spices: oregano, parsley, saffron, tarragon (all blend well with basic ingredients).
This recipe makes 1 pint of liquid.
Place all ingredients in a pint-sized jar. Shake vigorously to blend.

NOTE: With the T=T & T Diet, this dressing is suggested for all salads. The oils provided are vital to your system during your diet routine.

  * The above salad dressing was formulated by Julie and Frank Mackey of The Good Life Health Food Store of North Hollywood, California. The Mackeys' commonsense approach to healthful living inspires many who plan their entire daily menus around natural food stuffs. Learn to utilize your own local health food store, buying those preparations which particularly suit your own individual needs.

IDEAL WEIGHT*
Age 25 and over
Subtract 1 pound for each year under age 25
Weight in pounds according to frame
(in indoor clothing)

Height (with shoes on 2-inch heels)		Small frame	Medium frame	Large frame
Feet	Inches			
4	10	92- 98	96-107	104-119
4	11	94-101	98-110	106-122
5	0	96-104	101-113	109-125
5	1	99-107	104-116	112-128
5	2	102-110	107-119	115-131
5	3	105-113	110-122	118-134
5	4	108-116	113-126	121-138
5	5	111-119	116-130	125-142
5	6	114-123	120-135	129-146
5	7	118-127	124-139	133-150
5	8	122-131	128-143	137-154
5	9	126-135	132-147	141-158
5	10	130-140	136-151	145-163
5	11	134-144	140-155	149-168
6	0	138-148	144-159	153-173

* Statistics courtesy U. S. Department of Health, Education, and Welfare.

"DURABLE DYNAMO DIET" FOOD CHART

Including all those foods that meet four requirements:

1. Low in Calories
2. High in Protein
3. Low in Carbohydrate
4. Low in Saturated Fat

Food (one ounce or equivalent)	Calories	Protein	Carbo-hydrate	Saturated Fat
		(Stated in terms of grams per ounce unless otherwise described.)		
* Abalone	27	5.3	0.8	0.6
Artichokes (Globe)—⅓ cup	3	0.9	3.3	—
Asparagus (tips) —⅓ cup	3	0.7	1.2	—
Bamboo Shoots—½ large	9	0.9	1.7	—
* Bass	35	6.3	—	—
Beans, sprouted—½ cup	12	1.3	1.7	—
Beans, green—4 large	8	0.5	1.8	—
wax—4 large	7	0.5	1.5	—
* Beef, chuck	109	8.7	—	3.0
* flank steak	65	6.7	—	2.7
* round, trimmed	63	6.7	—	0.7
* ground, lean	73	9.1	—	1.7
dried, chipped—⅓ cup	68	11.4	—	1.0
Beet Greens—⅓ cup	8	0.7	1.5	—
* Bluefish	39	6.8	—	—
Bullion Cubes (1 cube)	3	0.4	0.1	—
* Brains	42	3.5	0.3	—
Broccoli—⅓ cup	9	1.0	1.5	—
Brussels Sprouts—⅓ cup	12	1.4	2.1	—
* Butterfish	32	5.4	—	—
Buttermilk—⅛ cup	12	1.3	1.7	1.0
Cabbage—2 leaves	8	0.4	1.8	—
Cantaloupe—⅛	10	0.2	2.5	—
* Carp	38	9.0	—	—
Cauliflower—⅓ cup	7	0.8	1.3	—
Celery (1 stalk) —⅓ cup	6	0.3	1.3	—
Chard—½ cup	6	0.9	1.1	—
Cheese				
Cottage, creamed—⅛ cup	36	4.5	0.9	0.9
uncreamed—⅛ cup	29	5.7	0.9	0.7

* For all items identified by (*) one ounce equals approximately one slice (1/8" thick, 4" long, 3" wide).

"DURABLE DYNAMO DIET" FOOD CHART

Food (one ounce or equivalent)	Calories	Protein	Carbo-hydrate	Saturated Fat
* Chicken, without skin	57	10.0	—	1.0
Chicken Consomme—⅛ cup	3	0.5	0.6	—
Chow mein (average)—¼ cup	34	3.1	1.3	0.3
Clams—6	33	5.3	0.6	—
* Cod	57	9.0	—	—
Coffee (black)	—	—	—	—
Coleslaw (made with safflower oil base) —¼ cup	43	0.4	1.7	0.3
Crab	31	5.8	0.2	—
Cucumber—4 slices	5	0.2	1.1	—
* Duck	55	7.1	—	—
Eggs—poached (one egg)	55	6.0	0.3	1.3
Eggplant—⅓ slice	6	0.3	1.7	—
Endive or Escarole— ½ small head	7	0.6	1.4	—
* Flounder	68	10.0	—	—
Frog Legs—2 small	24	5.5	—	—
Gizzards, chicken	38	6.7	0.2	—
* Goose	142	7.9	—	—
* Haddock	26	6.1	—	—
* Halibut	57	8.4	—	—
* Heart—beef	124	8.6	—	1.3
Herring, Pacific—⅓ small	33	5.8	—	0.7
Kale—⅓ cup	9	1.1	1.3	—
* Kidneys	84	11.0	0.3	—
* Lamb, leg	93	8.4	—	3.0
Lettuce—4 leaves	5	0.4	0.8	—
Lobster—¼ small	33	6.2	0.1	—
Milk, cow's fluid whole—⅛ cup	22	1.2	1.6	0.7
cow's fluid skim—⅛ cup	12	1.2	1.7	0.3
goat's fluid—⅛ cup	22	1.1	1.6	0.7
Mushrooms, fresh—⅓ cup	9	0.9	1.3	—
Mussels—6	22	3.2	1.0	—
Mustard Greens—¼ cup	10	1.0	1.8	—
Mustard, prepared—2 tbs.	30	1.9	1.8	—
New Zealand Spinach—¼ cup	4	0.4	0.7	—
Oils				
corn	250	—	—	3.3
cottonseed	250	—	—	8.3
olive	250	—	—	3.7
peanut	250	—	—	6.0
safflower	250	—	—	2.7
sesame	250	—	—	4.7
soybean	250	—	—	5.0
Olives (10 olives to oz.)	43	0.3	0.8	0.7

"DURABLE DYNAMO DIET" FOOD CHART

Food (one ounce or equivalent)	Calories	Protein	Carbo-hydrate	Saturated Fat
Onions, dry—¼ medium	33	0.5	2.9	—
Onions, green—2 small	32	0.5	2.9	—
Oysters (raw) 5 medium	22	2.8	2.8	1.1
Parsnips—¼ cup	22	0.5	5.0	—
Peppers, sweet—¼ medium	7	0.4	1.6	—
* Perch, Ocean	29	6.0	—	—
Pickles, dill—½ medium	4	0.2	0.7	—
* Pike	30	6.4	—	—
* Pompano	55	6.3	—	—
Protein Supplements				
Organ meats, desiccated, defatted & defibered				
Powder	112	26.0	—	—
Tablets—30	60	13.5	—	—
Liver, desiccated	124	17.0	2.3	7.0
Soy, Milk or Casein				
Mixtures (average)	110	9.5	14.1	1.0
Soybean (average)	110	19.3	5.0	1.0
Egg & Dry Milk (average)	110	17.0	7.2	1.0
* Rabbit	72	9.8	—	—
Radishes—4 medium	6	0.3	—	—
* Red Snapper	32	6.6	.—	—
* Rockfish	33	6.3	—	—
* Salmon	68	7.2	—	—
Sauerkraut Juice—⅛ cup	3	0.2	0.8	—
* Shad	67	7.8	—	—
Shrimp—2 large	30	6.0	0.5	—
* Smelt	33	6.2	—	—
Snails—4	30	5.4	0.7	—
**Soft drinks	—	—	—	—
* Sole	39	8.3	—	—
Squash, Summer—½ small	5	0.3	1.0	—
Yellow Crookneck—½ small	7	0.4	1.4	—
Zucchini—¼ small	6	0.4	1.2	—
Tea	—	—	—	—
Tomatoes—¼ medium	7	0.4	1.6	—
Tomato Juice—⅛ cup	6	0.3	1.4	—
* Tripe—pickled	31	4.0	—	—

** Dietetic Beverages: On the basis of a 12 fluid ounce bottle, there should be less than 1 calorie, no fat or protein, and less than ½ of 1% of available carbohydrates. Cheeck beverage labels. (Since cyclamates have been taken off the market, sugar content in low-cal drinks may be a trifle higher.)

"DURABLE DYNAMO DIET" FOOD CHART

Food (one ounce or equivalent)	Calories	Protein	Carbo-hydrate	Saturated Fat
* Trout	69	6.9	1.0	—
* Tuna (water packed)	43	9.3	0.3	—
* Turkey	88	9.0	1.3	1.3
Turnips—¼ cup	8	0.3	2.2	—
Turnip Greens—⅓ cup	7	0.7	1.2	—
* Veal—chuck	58	6.3	—	1.7
Watercress—20 sprigs	6	0.7	1.0	—
Yogurt—partially skim milk—⅛ cup	16	1.1	1.7	0.4

NOTE: Where foods are commonly eaten raw (lettuce, tomatoes, etc.) figures are given for raw. Wherever possible, when the common use is cooked, figures are given for the cooked product.

NOTE: The following sample diet menus may be followed for a week as an ideal example of how the DURABLE DYNAMO DIET works. In the future, you can make your own menus using the basic diet chart to figure out your calories, proteins, carbohydrates and saturated fats.

Following the seven sample menus, you will find a list of bonus foods which may be added once you have begun slimming down, or if you have a craving for something outside of the regular prescribed list. Please take care and do not over-indulge, or your bonus may turn into a booby-trap.

Make a selection from any of the foods on the chart. Caution:

CALORIES—not to exceed 600
CARBOHYDRATES—not to exceed 50 grams

These extras are to be added to totals on DYNAMO DIET

Foods	Calories	Carbo-hydrate Grams
TYPICAL BONUS DAY #1— 2 slices bread (can be used for sandwich)	160	32
½ orange	52	12.8
¼ cup sunflower seeds	200	2.8
TOTALS	412	47.6
TYPICAL BONUS DAY #2— 4 oz. macaroni and cheese	280	26.0
1 peach	60	16.0
¼ cup Brazil nuts	215	3.7
TOTALS	555	45.7
TYPICAL BONUS DAY #3— 3 scoops ice cream	207	20.7
¼ cup almonds	199	6.5
1 slice rye bread	82	17.5
TOTALS	488	44.7
TYPICAL BONUS DAY #4— fruit salad made of 1 apricot	394	48.9
10 grapes		
1 peach		
1 pear		
¼ cup sunflower seeds		
TOTALS	394	48.9
TYPICAL BONUS DAY #5— 1 roll	103	18.4
1 cup strawberries	48	11.2
2 cookies	100	15.4
TOTALS	251	45.0
TYPICAL BONUS DAY #6— 3" wedge apple pie	246	39.6
ala mode with 1 scoop ice cream	69	6.9
TOTALS	315	46.5

DURABLE DYNAMO DIET—SUGGESTED DIET #1

(in terms of grams per portion)

	Calories	Protein	Carbo-hydrate	Saturated Fats
BREAKFAST				
2 poached eggs	110	12.0	0.6	2.6
½ tomato (medium)	25	1.4	2.4	—
coffee or tea	—	—	—	—
LUNCH				
salad of				
½ head lettuce				
2 oz. tomatoes	76	5.0	14.0	—
2 oz. cucumbers				
2 oz. celery				
2 tbs. french dressing (safflower oil base)	120	—	4.0	2.0
4 oz. tuna (water pack)	172	37.2	1.2	—
coffee or tea	—	—	—	—
3:30 P.M.				
6 oz. cottage cheese (lightly creamed)	174	34.0	5.4	3.5
DINNER				
4 oz. coleslaw	172	1.6	6.8	1.2
⅓ lb. ground beef	389	48.0	—	9.0
*4 oz. cauliflower	28	3.2	5.2	—
4 oz. zucchini (cooked in beef cube)	27	2.0	4.9	—
SOMETIME DURING DAY				
1 tbs. good oil *(today's suggestion for use—steam cauliflower & then saute in oil)	125	—	—	1.3
DAILY TOTALS	1500	165	48	23

DURABLE DYNAMO DIET—SUGGESTED DIET #2

(in terms of grams per portion)

	Calories	Protein	Carbo-hydrate	Saturated Fats
BREAKFAST				
4 oz. ground beef	292	36.4	—	6.8
1 stalk celery	6	0.3	1.3	—
4 slices cucumber	5	0.2	1.1	—
coffee or tea	—	—	—	—
LUNCH				
5 oz. chicken (without the skin)	285	50.0	—	5.0
3 oz. cole slaw (dressing with safflower oil base)	120	1.2	5.1	0.9
coffee or tea	—	—	—	—
3:30 P.M.				
6 oz. buttermilk	72	7.8	10.2	6.0
DINNER				
5 oz. halibut	285	42.0	—	—
salad consisting of ½ sprigs watercress 4 slices tomato	62	4.7	11.4	—
2 tbs. French dressing (safflower oil base)	120	—	4.0	2.0
4 oz. broccoli (cook in beef cube)	31	4.4	6.1	—
*4 oz. green beans	32	2.0	5.0	—
coffee or tea	—	—	—	—
SOMETIME DURING DAY				
1 tbs. good oil	125	—	—	1.3
*(today's suggestion for use: after green beans are steamed tender, saute in oil and crushed garlic)				
DAILY TOTALS	1492	162.2	44.2	22

DURABLE DYNAMO DIET—SUGGESTED DIET #3

(in terms of grams per portion)

	Calories	Protein	Carbo-hydrate	Saturated Fat
BREAKFAST				
5 oz. salmon (water pack)	340	36.0	—	—
2 oz. green bell pepper	14	0.8	3.2	—
4 oz. tomato juice	24	1.2	5.6	—
coffee or tea	—	—	—	—
LUNCH				
*½ head lettuce	40	3.2	6.4	—
4 oz. herring	132	23.2	—	2.8
coffee or tea	—	—	—	—
3:30 P.M.				
3 oz. dried chipped beef	204	34.2	—	3.0
4 radishes	6	0.3	—	—
DINNER				
salad consisting of 6 oz. asparagus (canned or fresh)	18	4.2	7.2	—
2 tbs. French dressing	120	—	4.0	2.0
4 oz. turkey	352	36.0	5.2	3.9
*4 oz. spinach	16	1.6	2.8	—
4 oz. crookneck squash (cooked in bouillon cube)	31	2.0	5.6	—
coffee or tea	—	—	—	—
SOMETIME DURING DAY				
1 tbs. good oil	125	—	—	1.3
* (today's suggestion for use: use either as oil & vinegar dressing for lettuce at lunch or as oil and garlic dressing for spinach at dinner)				
DAILY TOTALS	1502	160	40	13

DURABLE DYNAMO DIET—SUGGESTED DIET #4

(in terms of grams per portion)

	Calories	Protein	Carbo-hydrate	Saturated Fat
BREAKFAST				
*2 eggs scrambled with	110	12.0	0.6	2.6
2 oz. fresh sliced mushrooms	18	1.8	2.6	—
4 oz. chopped tomatoes flavored with vegetable salt seasoning	28	1.6	6.4	—
coffee or tea	—	—	—	—
LUNCH				
salad consisting of				
¼ head lettuce	20	1.6	3.2	—
½ small zucchini chopped	8	0.6	3.6	—
12 sprigs watercress	6	0.7	1.0	—
3 oz. canned crab meat	93	17.4	0.6	—
2 tbs. French dressing (safflower oil base)	120	—	4.0	2.0
coffee or tea	—	—	—	—
3:30 P.M.				
5 oz. tuna (water pack)	215	46.5	1.5	—
½ tomato (medium)	25	1.4	2.4	—
2 oz. dill pickle	8	0.4	1.4	—
DINNER				
salad of 6 oz. cottage cheese (use low calorie Italian type dressing if desired)	216	27.0	5.4	5.4
4 oz. leg of lamb	372	33.6	—	12.0
4 oz. eggplant (cooked in beef or chicken cube)	24	1.2	6.8	—
4 oz. turnips	32	1.2	8.8	—
coffee or tea	—	—	—	—
SOMETIME DURING DAY				
1 tbs. good oil	125	—	—	1.3
* (today's suggestion for use: to scramble eggs)				
DAILY TOTALS	1500	165	48	23

DURABLE DYNAMO DIET—TYPICAL DIET #5

(in terms of grams per portion)

	Calories	Protein	Carbo-hydrate	Saturated Fat
BREAKFAST				
5 oz. breakfast round steak	315	33.5	—	3.5
2 stalks celery	12	0.6	2.6	—
coffee or tea	—	—	—	—
LUNCH				
crab salad of 7 oz. crab (average can)	217	40.6	1.4	—
⅓ cup celery	6	0.3	1.3	—
2 oz. yogurt as dressing	245	43.1	6.1	0.4
¼ cantaloupe—2 oz.	20	9.4	5.0	—
coffee or tea	—	—	—	—
3:30 P.M.				
8 oz. yogurt	128	8.8	11.9	3.2
2 oz. chipped dried beef	136	22.4	—	2.0
DINNER				
5 oysters on half shell	22	2.8	2.8	1.1
bell pepper stuffed with 4 oz. ground round and ⅓ cup celery	326	38.3	7.5	6.8
*broiled tomato (use oil and garlic)	28	1.6	5.6	—
*summer squash (2)	10	0.6	2.0	—
coffee or tea	—	—	—	—
SOMETIME DURING DAY				
1 tbs. good oil * (today's suggestion for use — divide between tomato and summer squash)	125	—	—	1.3
DAILY TOTALS	1427	165.3	43.5	18.3

DURABLE DYNAMO DIET—TYPICAL DIET #6

(in terms of grams per portion)

	Calories	Protein	Carbo-hydrate	Saturated Fat
BREAKFAST				
*omelet made with 2 eggs, 3 oz. chipped beef and ¼ cup green pepper	314	46.0	0.6	5.6
coffee or tea	—	—	—	—
LUNCH				
6 oz. cottage cheese	276	27.0	5.4	5.4
1 medium tomato	28	1.6	6.2	—
3:30 P.M.				
4 oz. chicken (cold)	228	40.0	—	—
DINNER				
salad of 5 oz. lobster ½ tomato 2 stalks celery 4 lettuce leaves	196	32.8	7.1	—
2 tbs. French dressing	120	—	4.0	2.0
6 oz. chow mein	204	12.4	5.2	1.2
coffee or tea	—	—	—	—
SOMETIME DURING DAY				
1 tbs. good oil	125	—	—	1.3
* (suggestion for today's use—use in omelet preparation)				
DAILY TOTALS	1498	173.8	30.1	15.5

DURABLE DYNAMO DIET—TYPICAL DIET #7

(in terms of grams per portion)

	Calories	Protein	Carbo-hydrate	Saturated Fat
BREAKFAST				
5 oz. yogurt	80	5.5	8.5	2.0
1 medium tomato	28	1.6	6.2	—
coffee or tea	—	—	—	—
LUNCH				
1 cup coleslaw	172	1.6	6.8	1.2
8 oz. filet of sole	312	66.4	—	—
coffee or tea	—	—	—	—
3:30 P.M.				
lettuce-lamb sandwich 3 oz. cold lamb wrapped in lettuce leaf)	280	25.2	0.2	9.0
DINNER				
salad of 3 oz. cottage cheese, 1 lettuce leaf 12 sprigs chopped watercress, 1 oz. chopped green onion	159	19.3	7.7	3.6
4 oz. roast veal	232	25.2	—	6.8
*1 cup chard	12	1.8	2.2	—
*1 cup turnips	32	1.2	4.4	—
coffee or tca	—	—	—	—
SOMETIME DURING DAY				
1 tbs. good oil * (suggestion for today's use—on turnips and chard with seasonings)	125	—	—	1.3
DAILY TOTALS	1492	161.0	36.0	23.9

BONUS FOODS CHART

FRUITS	1 oz. Equals Approx.	Calories	Carbohydrates
Blackberries	¼ cup	19	4.1
Blueberries	¼ cup	20	4.3
Raspberries	¼ cup	19	4.6
Strawberries	¼ cup	12	2.8
Grapefruit	1 section	13	3.2
Oranges	1 section	15	3.8
Honey Dew Melon	5 balls	11	2.8
Watermelon	5 balls	9	2.3
Apples	¼ small	28	5.0
Apricots	1 small	27	4.3
Grapes	10 seedless	23	5.0
Guavas	½ small	23	5.7
Peaches	¼ medium	15	4.0
Pears	¼ small	21	5.2
Plums	½ medium	17	4.3

FRUIT JUICES

Apple Juice	⅛ cup	17	4.4
Grape Juice	⅛ cup	22	6.1
Grapefruit Juice	⅛ cup	18	4.4
Orange Juice	⅛ cup	15	3.7
Pineapple Juice	⅛ cup	15	4.3
Tomato Juice	⅛ cup	7	1.4

BREADS & BAKED PRODUCTS

Whole Wheat Bread	1 slice	80	16.0
Rye Bread	1 slice	82	17.5
White Bread	1 slice	92	17.9
Angel Food Cake	2" slice	90	19.5
Corn Bread	1 small muffin	73	12.2
Macaroni & Cheese	2 tbs.	70	6.5
Muffins	1 small	93	14.0
Pancakes	1 medium	73	8.9
Apple Pie	1" wedge 8" pie	82	13.2
Rolls (plain)	1 small	103	18.4
Cookies (average)	3 small	150	23.0

NUTS

Almonds	¼ cup	199	6.5
Brazils	¼ cup	215	3.7
Cashews	¼ cup	193	9.0
Pecans	¼ cup	232	5.2
Sunflower Seeds	¼ cup (scant)	200	2.8
Filberts	¼ cup	211	5.6
Pumpkin Seeds	¼ cup (scant)	184	5.0

MISCELLANEOUS

Ice Cream	1 small scoop	69	6.9
Sherbert	1 small scoop	41	10.0

"T = T & T"

CHAPTER FOURTEEN

In the year 1866, Alfred Nobel discovered dynamite.
This discovery paved the way for a whole series of explosives. Everyone knows the symbol "T.N.T.", which actually stands for the word *trinitrotoluene* and has come to be used commonly as a symbol to describe any explosive force.

More than a hundred years later, we have come upon a new "beauty formula" which is written:

$$T = T \; \& \; T$$

In this case, the symbolic letters add up to *potentially potent personal dynamite!* "Playing the Beauty Game" successfully is assured when you follow this diet plan.

> T — Thirty Days
>   equals
> T — Twenty pounds off
>   and
> T — Ten years younger looking

Could anything be more simple? Our "beauty formula" is as uncomplicated and basic as the ABC's. It works on the very same principle. First, you have to learn the "formula"; then you have to begin to use it. Eventually, it becomes an automatic part of your daily life. Both "formulas" actually are fundamental tools created to enable you to go through life more successfully. The ABC's are your means of communicating. $T = T \& T$ is a formula which will lead you toward projecting the most lovely image possible.

This chapter contains one specially formulated diet which has been designed for MAXIMUM weight loss with a MINIMUM amount of effort. You will feel no starvation pangs, and what's more you will have enough energy to keep you going—hunger free and happy.

Prior to going into the specifics of this new "beauty formula," we must caution you. Before undertaking any diet, a physical check-up with your own physician is a must. Tell your doctor you wish to try this diet. Show it to him. Discuss it with him. Do NOT proceed until he has given you the green light to begin.

Once you have ascertained that you are in fit physical condition to begin this new regimen, first study the diet and supplementary explanations very carefully. Be sure you understand what it is we are aiming to help you accomplish. Do NOT go rushing off pell mell in your enthusiasm to begin. If you have had a weight problem for any length of time, and you are now serious about wishing to get rid of your excessive poundage for GOOD, there is no reason to rush headlong into anything until you really understand where you are going and exactly how you are going to get there!

This $T = T \& T$ "beauty formula" can be the beginning of a new life for you. If you follow the directions carefully, in thirty days you can lose twenty pounds, look ten years younger, and FEEL ten years younger, too.

WORDS OF CAUTION BEFORE STARTING ON THE T = T & T ROUTINE:

1. Each day, for thirty days, your breakfast, lunch and dinner has been mathematically computed. There can be NO deviations, as any would throw off the arithmetic balance. There is only *one* change which you *can* make if you desire. You can switch the SEQUENCE of meals within any one given day. For instance, if you want to switch the breakfast menu of Day #1 with the lunch menu for Day #1 this is fine. But you *cannot* switch breakfast of Day #1 with say lunch of Day #3. NO SWITCHING OF MENUS EXCEPT WITHIN THE SAME DAY.

2. You will see that each day's menu contains the word SNACK at the bottom. This indicates the *only other* food intake allowable within that given day. You should take your snack *no later than four o'clock in the afternoon* on any given day. Or, you may choose to include your snack allowance *within* your breakfast, lunch, or dinner. You *cannot* carry it over to the next day's meals. It must be consumed on the day upon which it was scheduled.

3. There can be NO substitution of one meat for the other, one vegetable or fruit for another, etc. Each element of the thirty days' diet has a special meaning. To be most effective, it must be utilized when it is scheduled.

4. All meats listed should be lean, with any excess fat trimmed away PRIOR to cooking. Meats may be broiled, baked, pan broiled only. Do NOT fry any foods unless otherwise indicated.

5. All chicken and turkey should be served *with the skin removed.*

6. Each day you *must* have a certain amount of a good oil in your diet. You will note that on days when the oil is not already provided for within the menus, suggestions are made about cooking various vegetables in oil. DO THIS. Use any good oil, among which are safflower oil, sesame seed oil, corn oil.

*7. Beverages such as coffee and tea are to be taken WITHOUT CREAM AND SUGAR. Where you wish, coffee or tea may be deleted provided you substitute a low calorie-type beverage. On the basis of a 12 fluid ounce bottle, there should be very few calories, no fat or protein, and less than ½ of one percent of available carbohydrates. Check this information on individual beverage bottle labels.

8. You will note that each meal of every day's menu lists a "PROTEIN SUPPLEMENT". *This is essential.* The protein supplement you select (in tablet or powdered form) must be a supplement derived from organ meats, dessicated, defatted and defibered. Your doctor, druggist, or health food store proprietor can help you select the proper type of protein supplement. Do NOT eliminate this—it is ESSENTIAL to the overall success of the T = T & T formula.

9. You will note our suggestions of other things to be done in concert with the diet menus. You will find suggestions for an exercise time, a brisk walking period, a facial, pedicure, hair care treatment, etc. THESE ARE OPTIONAL and may be used or not, as YOU wish. They can also be switched from day to day and sequence to sequence. These have been listed merely as GUIDELINES. It is up to you to make your own personal schedule for employing beauty rituals to

---

* You may want to carefully utilize low-calorie sugar and milk substitutes found on the market. Do so with caution!

suit your own personal needs and time. NOTE: Recipes for all facials, shampoos, etc., will be found in Chapter 30 under "Do-It-Yourself Cosmetics".

10. It is suggested that you study the menus, make a list of food needed for a week at a time, or a few days at a time where foodstuffs spoil rapidly. Buy food for at least three days in advance so you are always sure to have the exact menus on hand. Since deviation from set menus lessens the effectiveness of the diet, it is ESSENTIAL that you plan your menus ahead of time.

11. Note: Where fruits such as strawberries are listed, these are to be *fresh* fruits or, if necessary, canned of the *water-packed* variety. Do NOT use any fruits in heavy syrup. Be sure to rinse all water-packed fruit so it is as free from juice as possible. If you do have to use canned fruits, cut the amount specified in half to insure that you stay within the proscribed mathematical balance we have worked out for you.

Now that you have read all our words of caution, we should add a few more words—of ENCOURAGEMENT.

There is no reason why you cannot lose weight on this diet. Unless you are one of that rare breed whose obesity stems from more than plain over-eating, this specially formulated diet should work, provided you follow it to the letter, and DO NOT cheat!

There is NO reason to "go off the wagon" with this diet. You will NOT feel the least bit hungry while you are on it. You will have NO craving for sweets. But remember, unless you really are serious about trying to follow the T = T & T "beauty formula" to the letter, don't bother to begin. This diet routine will NOT work if you make any substitutions other than those specified as permissible.

After you have your own doctor's permission to begin, start this exciting new plan as soon as possible.

You have nothing to lose but your bulges! Besides, we know from hundreds of comments already received, from many calls and letters we have examined, that once you are on this diet you WILL look better and FEEL better and function BETTER.

Don't say we didn't warn you: $T = T \,\&\, T$ may very well become as important to your way of life as your basic ABC's! In any event, the more you work for self-improvement, the more opportunity you'll have to share in the fun made possible when you "Play the Beauty Game" to the fullest extent!

Only Thirty Days to Go!

CHAPTER FIFTEEN

In preceding chapters, we discussed the fundamentals of the type of diet which now follows. We cannot stress too strongly the preparations which you must take *before* embarking on this regimen. See your personal physician FIRST. Show him the diet. Allow him to make the decision as to whether or not you are physically able to go on this diet. Once you have his blessings, begin!

Again, let me advise you to go through the daily menus until you have familiarized yourself with the over-all pattern. Make a list of the foods you'll need for the first week. Shop wisely and get all the supplies in before you begin.

Set a weight loss goal for yourself. Decide realistically how much you want to lose. Remember: you didn't get those hip and thigh bulges overnight. It will take MORE than overnight to eliminate them.

Put your mind at ease. Don't start this diet plan if you are under an unusually severe strain. Cheating— even a little bit—can be a disaster on a diet which is mathematically formulated. Better to wait until you are in a good frame of mind before you begin. Be fair to yourself—start with all the advantages on your side.

Remember, T = T & T is NOT a magic formula. But it CAN and WILL work if followed correctly. And now, assuming you have made all necessary preparations—BEGIN and be prepared to see a new you emerging!

FIRST DAY—#1

EXERCISE—10 MINUTES

BREAKFAST

5 ounces	Tuna (water packed)
1/2 medium	Tomato
	Coffee or tea
	Protein supplement

BRISK WALK

LUNCH

4 ounces	Leg of lamb
1/3 cup	Cauliflower**
1/4 cup	Strawberries
	Coffee or tea
	Protein supplement

EXERCISE—15 MINUTES

DINNER

5 ounces	Halibut
4 ounces	Green beans
5 balls	Honey dew melon
	Coffee or tea
	Protein supplement

BATH—"DAYDREAMERS"

**Cooked in 1 tbs. oil

SNACK—4 large shrimp
　　　　4 ounces cole slaw

SECOND DAY—#2

EXERCISE—15 minutes

BREAKFAST

2	Poached eggs
½ medium	Tomato
	Coffee or tea
	Protein supplement

FACIAL "LOVER'S LOTION"

LUNCH

8 ounces	Filet of sole
1 medium	Tomato (broiled) **
6 ounces	Buttermilk (or coffee or tea)
	Protein supplement

BRISK WALK

DINNER

4 ounces	Roast veal
1 cup	Cole slaw
¼ section	Cantaloupe
	Coffee or tea
	Protein supplement

PEDICURE

**Cooked with 1 tbs. oil

SNACK—1 tomato
  1 cup of chow mein

THIRD DAY—#3

HAIR TREATMENT

BREAKFAST

5 ounces	Cube steak
⅓ cup	Asparagus tips
	Coffee or tea
	Protein supplement

Third Day #3 (*continued*)

EXERCISE—20 minutes
LUNCH
4 ounces	Turkey
1/3 cup	Broccoli
1/4 portion	Cantaloupe
	Coffee or tea
	Protein supplement

DINNER
1/8 cup	Grape juice
	(fill glass with iced water)
	Omelet
	with
2	Eggs
3 ounces	Chipped beef
1/4 cup	Green peppers
	Salad
	with
1/2 head	Lettuce
1/2 medium	Tomato
4 slices	Cucumber
2 stalks	Celery
2 tbs.	French dressing
	Coffee or tea
	Protein supplement

BATH "LIME TONIC"
FACIAL "LOVER'S LOTION"
SNACK—3 large shrimp
        4 ounces cole slaw

FOURTH DAY—#4
BRISK WALK
BREAKFAST
1/2	Medium tomato
5 ounces	Breakfast round steak
4 slices	Cucumber
	Coffee or tea
	Protein supplement

Fourth Day #4 (*continued*)
FACIAL "DEBUTANTE'S DELIGHT"
    LUNCH
      2   Scrambled eggs
                                    with
      2 ounces   Fresh sliced mushrooms
      ⅓ cup   Brussels sprouts
      6 ounces   Buttermilk (or coffee or tea)
                                    Protein supplement

EXERCISE—15 MINUTES
    DINNER
                                  Lobster salad
                                  with
      5 ounces   Lobster
      ½ medium   Tomato
      2 stalks   Celery
      ¼ head   Lettuce
      2 Tbs.   French Dressing
                                    Coffee or tea
                                  Protein supplement
      1 small   Sherbet
        scoop

MANICURE—OIL

SNACK—4 ounces cold chicken
        ½ small dill pickle

FIFTH DAY—#5

EXERCISE—15 minutes
    BREAKFAST
      4 ounces   Ground Beef Patty
      4 slices   Cucumber
                                    Coffee or tea
                                  Protein supplement

    LUNCH
      1 cup   Tomato juice
                                  Salad
      2 Tbs.   with French dressing
      6 ounces   Cottage cheese
                                    (lightly creamed)

Fifth Day #5 (*continued*)

4	Radishes
2	Celery stalks
4	Cucumber slices
	Coffee or tea
	Protein supplement

SIESTA—15 minutes
    DINNER

⅛ cup	Apple juice
	(fill glass with iced water)
⅓ pound	Ground Beef
4 ounces	Broccoli
1 cup	Cole slaw
	Coffee or tea
	Protein supplement

EXERCISE—20 minutes

FACIAL "JET SET SPECIAL"

SNACK—4 large shrimp
      ½ tomato

SIXTH DAY—#6

BRISK WALK
    BREAKFAST

2	Scrambled eggs
½ medium	Tomato
	Coffee or tea
	Protein supplement

    LUNCH

3 ounces	Cold lamb slices
½ cup	Broccoli**
½ cup	Sliced apples
	Coffee or tea
	Protein supplement

EXERCISE—15 MINUTES
    DINNER

⅛ cup	Pineapple juice
	(fill glass with iced water)
5 ounces	Chicken (no skin)
4 ounces	Zucchini**

**Cooked with 1 tbs. oil

Sixth Day #6 *(continued)*

4 ounces	Green beans
	Coffee and tea
	Protein supplement

BEAUTY RITUAL:
 FACIAL "DEBUTANTE'S DELIGHT"

 BATH "PARISIAN AROMATIC"

SNACK—4 ounces chicken
 ½ dill pickle

SEVENTH DAY—#7

EXERCISE—15 MINUTES
 BREAKFAST

5 ounces	Breakfast round steak
4 slices	Cucumber
½ medium	Tomato
	Coffee or tea
	Protein supplement

 LUNCH

4 ounces	Leg of lamb
⅓ cup	Cauliflower
¼ cup	Strawberries
	Coffee or tea
	Protein supplement

BRISK WALK
 DINNER

4 ounces	Roast veal
	Salad
	with
¼ head	Lettuce
½ medium	Tomato
4 slices	Cucumber
2 stalks	Celery
2 Tbs.	French dressing
½ cup	Sherbet
	Coffee or tea
	Protein supplement

Seventh Day #7 (*continued*)
BEAUTY RITUAL:
    FACIAL MASQUE "SUNNY SIDE UP"
    SHAMPOO—HAIR CARE TREATMENT
SNACK—4 ounces tuna (water packed)
       ½ dill pickle

EIGHTH DAY—#8

BREAKFAST

5 ounces	Tuna (water packed)
½ medium	Tomato
	Coffee or tea
	Protein supplement

BRISK WALK
LUNCH

	with
2 Tbs.	French dressing
6 ounces	Cottage cheese
	(lightly creamed)
4	Radishes
2 stalks	Celery
4 slices	Cucumber
1 cup	Tomato juice
	Coffee or tea
	Protein supplement

PROFESSIONAL MASSAGE
DINNER

⅛ cup	Apple juice
	(fill glass with iced water)
⅓ pound	Ground beef patty
4 ounces	Broccoli
1 cup	Cole slaw
	Coffee or tea
	Protein supplement

EXERCISE—30 MINUTES—
BATH "TROPICAL TEMPTATION"

SNACK—1 cup chow mein

NINTH DAY—#9

EXERCISE—15 MINUTES
BREAKFAST

2	Scrambled eggs
½ medium	Tomato
	Coffee or tea
	Protein supplement

BRISK WALK
LUNCH

	Lobster Salad
	with
5 ounces	Lobster
½ medium	Tomato
2 stalks	Celery
¼ head	Lettuce
2 Tbs.	French Dressing
1 small scoop	Sherbet
	Coffee or tea
	Protein supplement

DINNER

4 ounces	Roast veal
1 cup	Cole slaw
¼ portion	Cantaloupe
	Coffee or tea
	Protein supplement

EXERCISE AND BEAUTY RITUAL:
FACIAL "PAPAYA PAQUE"
BATH "ROMAN ROSE"

SNACK—3 ounces cold chicken
1 tomato broiled with 1 tbs. oil

TENTH DAY—#10

EXERCISE—15 MINUTES
BREAKFAST

5 ounces	Cube steak
⅓ cup	Asparagus tips**
	Coffee or tea
	Protein supplement

Tenth Day #10 *(continued)*

LUNCH

8 ounces	Filet of Sole
1 medium	Tomato
6 ounces	Buttermilk (or coffee or tea)
	Protein supplement

BRISK WALK

DINNER

⅛ cup	Pineapple juice (fill glass with iced water)
5 ounces	Chicken (no skin)
4 ounces	Zucchini**
⅓ cup	Green beans
	Coffee or tea
	Protein supplement

BEAUTY RITUAL: FACIAL "BASIC BUTTERMILK"

**Cooked with 1 tbs. oil

SNACK—1 cup chow mein

ELEVENTH DAY—#11

BRISK WALK

BREAKFAST

4 ounces	Ground beef patty
4 slices	Cucumber
	Coffee or tea
	Protein supplement

LUNCH

5 ounces	Tuna (water packed)
½ medium	Tomato
4 slices	Cucumber
	Coffeee or tea
	Protein supplement

EXERCISE—15 MINUTES

DINNER

⅛ cup	Grape juice (fill glass with iced water)
	Omelet with
2	Eggs
3 ounces	Chipped beef

Eleventh Day #11 (*continued*)

¼ cup	Green peppers
	Salad
	with
½ head	Lettuce
½ medium	Tomato
4 slices	Cucumber
2 stalks	Celery
2 tbs.	French dressing
	Coffee or tea
	Protein supplement

EXERCISE AND BEAUTY RITUAL:
FACIAL PACK "JET SET SPECIAL"
SNACK—4 large shrimp
　　　3 ounces cole slaw

TWELFTH DAY—#12

EXERCISE—15 MINUTES
　BREAKFAST

2	Poached eggs
½ medium	Tomato
	Coffee or tea
	Protein supplement

EXERCISE—15 MINUTES
　LUNCH

4 ounces	Turkey
⅓ cup	Broccoli**
¼ portion	Cantaloupe
	Coffee or tea
	Protein supplement

BRISK WALK
　DINNER

5 ounces	Halibut
4 ounces	Green beans**
5 balls	Honey dew melon
	Coffee or tea
	Protein supplement

RELAXING BATH "DAY DREAMERS"
FACIAL MASQUE "EAST INDIAN HERBAL"
　　　　　　　　　**Cooked with 1 tbs. oil

SNACK—8 ounces yogurt
　　　1 slice lamb

THIRTEENTH DAY—#13

EXERCISE—15 MINUTES
    BREAKFAST

	Omelet
	with
2	Eggs
3 ounces	Chopped green peppers
1 medium	Tomato
2 stalks	Celery
	Coffee or tea
	Protein supplement

SAUNA STEAM BATH AND HAIR TREATMENT
    LUNCH

5 ounces	Salmon (water packed)
4 ounces	Spinach
½ medium	Tomato
½ small	Apple
	Coffee or tea
	Protein supplement

BRISK WALK
    DINNER

5 ounces	Round Steak
½ small head	Lettuce
4	Radishes
½ medium	Tomato
2 Tbs.	French Dressing
⅛ cup	Grape juice
	(fill glass with iced water)
	Protein supplement
	Coffee or tea

BRISK WALK AND BEAUTY RITUAL:
FACIAL MASQUE "MILKMAID'S JEWELS"
SNACK—4 ounces chicken
    ½ dill pickle

FOURTEENTH DAY—#14

EXERCISE—15 MINUTES
    BREAKFAST

5 ounces	Chicken (without skin)
½ medium	Tomato
	Coffee or tea
	Protein supplement

Fourteenth Day #14 (*continued*)
FACIAL "HOT SCOTCH"
    LUNCH

4 ounces	Leg of lamb
4 ounces	Cole slaw
1 medium	Tomato
¼ portion	Cantaloupe
	Coffee or tea
	Protein supplement

BRISK WALK
    DINNER

⅓ pound	Ground beef patty
½ cup	Green beans**
⅓ cup	Asparagus tips**
1 tiny bunch	Seedless grapes
(15 to 20)	
	Coffee or tea
	Protein supplement

PEDICURE AND MANICURE

                       **Cooked with 1 tbs. oil

SNACK—4 large shrimp
       ½ tomato

FIFTEENTH DAY—#15

BRISK WALK AND FACIAL "BASIC BUTTERMILK
MASQUE"
    BREAKFAST

2	Poached eggs
½ medium	Tomato
	Coffee or tea
	Protein supplement

    LUNCH

1 small	Bell pepper
	stuffed with
4 ounces	Ground round
⅓ cup	Chopped celery
4 ounces	Tomato juice
½ small	Apple
	Coffee or tea
	Protein supplement

Fifteenth Day #15 (*continued*)
SIESTA—15 MINUTES
    DINNER

1 cup	Cole slaw
4 ounces	Flounder broiled with: 2 Tbs. oil and:
1 medium	Tomato
⅓ cup	Mushrooms
2 stalks	Celery
½ small	Apple
	Coffee or tea
	Protein supplement

EXERCISE 20 MINUTES AND BATH "ROMAN ROSE"

SNACK—3 ounces of chicken (without skin)

SIXTEENTH DAY—#16

EXERCISE—20 MINUTES
    BREAKFAST

4 ounces	Ground beef patty
4 slices	Cucumber
	Coffee or tea
	Protein supplement

    LUNCH

5 ounces	Chicken (without skin)
1 cup	Cole slaw
3 ounces	Chow mein
	Coffee or tea
	Protein supplement

BRISK WALK
    DINNER

4 ounces	Turkey (without skin)
2 small	Summer squash**
1 slice	Whole wheat toast (dry)
½ small	Apple
	Coffee or tea
	Protein supplement

BEAUTY RITUAL: BATH "ROSE WATER"
AND FACIAL PACK "OOH-LA-LA"

                                     **cook in 1 tbs. oil.

SNACK: 4 large shrimp
        ½ tomato broiled in 1 tbs. oil

SEVENTEENTH DAY—#17

BRISK WALK

BREAKFAST

2	Scrambled eggs
½ medium	Tomato
	Coffee or tea
	Protein supplement

LUNCH

	Seafood salad
	with
5 ounces	Lobster
4 small	Shrimp
2 ounces	Crab
½ medium	Tomato
2 stalks	Celery
2 tbs.	French dressing
	Coffee or tea
	Protein supplement

EXERCISE—15 MINUTES

DINNER

4 ounces	Roast veal
1 cup	Cole slaw
¼ portion	Cantaloupe
	Coffee or tea
	Protein supplement

BRISK WALK AND BEAUTY RITUAL:
FACIAL SAUNA AND BATH "DAY DREAMERS"

SNACK: 4 ounces chicken (without skin)
　　　　½ dill pickle

EIGHTEENTH DAY—#18

EXERCISE—20 MINUTES

BREAKFAST

2	Poached eggs
½ medium	Tomato
	Coffee or tea
	Protein supplement

Eighteenth Day #18 (*continued*)

LUNCH

4 ounces	Roast veal
1 cup	Cole slaw
1/4 portion	Cantaloupe
	Coffee or tea
	Protein supplement

BRISK WALK AND FACIAL "MOON GLOW"

DINNER

8 ounces	Filet of sole
1 medium	Broiled tomato**
6 ounces	Buttermilk
	(or coffee or tea)
	Protein supplement

**Cook with 1 tbs. oil

SNACK: 4 large shrimp
        4 ounces cole slaw

NINETEENTH DAY—#19

EXERCISE—15 MINUTES

BREAKFAST

5 ounces	Tuna (water packed)
1/2 medium	Tomato
	Coffee or tea
	Protein supplement

BRISK WALK

LUNCH

1/8 cup	Apple juice (fill glass with iced water)
1/3 pound	Ground beef patty
4 ounces	Cole slaw
1 cup	Broccoli**
	Coffee or tea
	Protein supplement

EXERCISE—15 MINUTES

**Cook with 1 tbs. oil

Nineteenth Day #19 (*continued*)
    DINNER

	Salad
2 tbs.	French Dressing
6 ounces	Cottage cheese (lightly creamed)
4	Radishes
2 stalks	Celery
4 slices	Cucumber
1 cup	Tomato juice
	Coffee or tea
	Protein supplement

EXERCISE AND BEAUTY RITUAL—"GOING NATIVE"
SNACK: 3 large shrimp
      ½ tomato

TWENTIETH DAY—#20

    BREAKFAST

5 ounces	Chicken (without skin)
4 ounces	Zucchini**
⅓ cup	Green beans**
	Coffee or tea
	Protein supplement

EXERCISE—15 MINUTES
    LUNCH

⅛ cup	Pineapple juice (fill glass with iced water)
5 ounces	Cube steak
⅓ cup	Asparagus tips
	Coffee or tea
	Protein supplement

BRISK WALK
    DINNER

8 ounces	Filet of sole
1 medium	Tomato
6 ounces	Buttermilk (or coffee or tea)
	Protein supplement

BEAUTY RITUAL—PEDICURE and
FACIAL "EGGS-BEES-VEE'S"

                            **Cook with 1 tbs. oil

SNACK: 4 large shrimp
      ½ tomato

TWENTY-FIRST DAY—#21

BREAKFAST

5 ounces	Tuna (water packed)
½ medium	Tomato
4 slices	Cucumber
	Coffee or tea
	Protein supplement

LUNCH

4 ounces	Ground beef patty
4 slices	Cucumber
	Coffee or tea
	Protein supplement

EXERCISE—20 MINUTES

DINNER

⅛ cup	Grape juice (fill glass with iced water)
	Omelet with:
2	Eggs
3 ounces	Chipped beef
¼ cup	Green peppers
	Salad with:
½ head	Lettuce
½ medium	Tomato
4 slices	Cucumber
2 stalks	Celery
2 tbs.	French Dressing
	Coffee or tea
	Protein supplement

**BRISK WALK AND BEAUTY RITUAL:
FACIAL MASQUE "HINT OF MINT"**

SNACK: 5 ounces yogurt
1 slice lamb

TWENTY-SECOND DAY—#22

EXERCISE—15 MINUTES

BREAKFAST

5 balls	Honey dew melon
5 ounces	Halibut**
4 ounces	Green beans
	Coffee or tea
	Protein supplement

Twenty-Second Day #22 (*continued*)

LUNCH

2	Poached eggs
1/2 medium	Tomato
	Coffee or tea
	Protein supplement

BRISK WALK

DINNER

4 ounces	Turkey (without skin)
1/3 cup	Broccoli**
1/4 portion	Cantaloupe
	Coffee or tea
	Protein supplement

EXERCISE—20 MINUTES AND BEAUTY RITUAL: BATH "PARISIAN AROMATIC"

**cook with 1 tbs. oil

SNACK: 4 ounces yogurt
      1 slice lamb

TWENTY-THIRD DAY—#23

BRISK WALK

BREAKFAST

5 ounces	Tuna (water packed)
1/2 medium	Tomato
	Coffee or tea
	Protein supplement

LUNCH

5 ounces	Halibut
4 ounces	Green beans**
5 balls	Honey dew melon
	Coffee or tea
	Protein supplement

EXERCISE—20 MINUTES

DINNER

4 ounces	Leg of lamb
1/3 cup	Cauliflower**
1/4 cup	Strawberries
	Coffee or tea
	Protein supplement

Twenty-Third Day #23 (*continued*)

BRISK WALK AND BEAUTY RITUAL:
FACIAL "A LA CREME"
AND BOTH "TROPICAL TEMPTATION"

**Cook with 1 tbs. oil

SNACK: 4 shrimp
4 ounces cole slaw

TWENTY-FOURTH DAY—#24

EXERCISE—15 MINUTES

BREAKFAST

2	Scrambled eggs with:
2 ounces	Fresh sliced mushrooms
1/3 cup	Brussels sprouts**
6 ounces	Buttermilk (or coffee or tea)
	Protein supplement

BRISK WALK

LUNCH

1/2 medium	Tomato
5 ounces	Round steak
4 slices	Cucumber coffee or tea
	Protein supplement

EXERCISE—15 MINUTES

DINNER

	Lobster Salad with:
5 ounces	Lobster
1/2 medium	Tomato
2 stalks	Celery
1/4 head	Lettuce
2 tbs.	French dressing
1 small scoop	Sherbert
	Coffee or tea
	Protein supplement

PEDICURE AND FACIAL "NUTS TO YOU"

**Cook with 1 tbs. oil

SNACK: 3 ounces chicken
1/2 dill pickle

TWENTY-FIFTH DAY—#25

BREAKFAST

2	Scrambled eggs
½ medium	Tomato
	Coffee or tea
	Protein supplement

BRISK WALK AND EXERCISE—25 MINUTES

LUNCH

⅛ cup	Pineapple juice (fill glass with iced water)
5 ounces	Chicken (without skin)
4 ounces	Zucchini**
4 ounces	Green beans
	Coffee and tea
	Protein supplement

HAIR CARE TREATMENT

DINNER

3 ounces	Cold lamb slices
½ cup	Broccoli**
½ cup	Sliced apples
	Coffee or tea
	Protein supplement

SHAMPOO WITH ACID MANTLE AID AND FACIAL SAUNA

SNACK: 4 ounces cottage cheese (lightly creamed)

**Cook with 1 tbs. oil

½ tomato
2 stalks celery

TWENTY-SIXTH DAY—#26

BRISK WALK

BREAKFAST

4 ounces	Leg of lamb
⅓ cup	Cauliflower**
¼ cup	Strawberries
	Coffee or tea
	Protein supplement

Twenty-Sixth Day #26 (*continued*)

EXERCISE—10 MINUTES

LUNCH

5 ounces	Round steak
4 slices	Cucumber
½ medium	Tomato
	Coffee or tea
	Protein supplement

EXERCISE—15 MINUTES

DINNER

4 ounces	Roast veal
	Salad with:
½ head	Lettuce
½ medium	Tomato
4 slices	Cucumber
2 stalks	Celery
2 Tbs.	French dressing
½ cup	Sherbet
	Coffee or tea
	Protein supplement

EXERCISE—20 MINUTES

**Cook with 1 tbs. oil

SNACK: 5 ounces yogurt
         1 slice lamb

TWENTY-SEVENTH DAY—#27

BRISK WALK

BREAKFAST

2	Scrambled eggs
½ medium	Tomato
	Coffee or tea
	Protein supplement

FACIAL "LOVER'S LOTION"

LUNCH

	Lobster salad with:
5 ounces	Lobster
½ medium	Tomato
2 stalks	Celery

Twenty-Seventh Day #27 (*continued*)

½ head	Lettuce
2 tbs.	French dressing
1 small scoop	Sherbet
	Coffee or tea
	Protein supplement

BRISK WALK

DINNER

4 ounces	Roast veal
1 cup	Green Beans**
¼ portion	Cantaloupe
	Coffee or tea
	Protein supplement

EXERCISE—15 MINUTES AND BEAUTY RITUAL:
BATH "TROPICAL TEMPTATION"

**Cook with 1 tbs. oil

SNACK: 5 ounces chicken (without skin)
½ tomato

TWENTY-EIGHTH DAY—#28

EXERCISE—15 MINUTES

BREAKFAST

5 ounces	Chicken (without skin)
½ medium	Tomato
	Coffee or tea
	Protein supplement

LUNCH

⅓ pound	Ground beef patty
½ cup	Green beans**
⅓ cup	Asparagus tips
1 tiny bunch (15 to 20)	Seedless grapes
	Coffee or tea
	Protein supplement

BRISK WALK

DINNER

4 ounces	Leg of lamb
4 ounces	Cole slaw

Twenty-Eighth Day #28 (*continued*)

1 medium	Tomato
1/4 portion	Cantaloupe
	Coffee or tea
	Protein supplement

EXERCISE—15 MINUTES AND
BEAUTY RITUAL: MANICURE & PEDICURE

**Cook with 1 tbs. oil

SNACK: 4 ounces tuna (water packed)
1/2 tomato

TWENTY-NINTH DAY—#29

BREAKFAST

2	Poached eggs
1/2 medium	Tomato
	Coffee or tea
	Protein supplement

EXERCISE AND BRISK WALK—

30 MINUTES COMBINED

LUNCH

1 cup	Cole slaw
4 ounces	Flounder (broiled) with:
1 medium	Tomato
1/3 cup	Mushrooms**
2 stalks	Celery
1/2 small	Apple
	Coffee or tea
	Protein supplement

FACIAL "LOVER'S LOTION"

DINNER

1 small	Bell pepper stuffed with:
4 ounces	Ground round
1/3 cup	Chopped celery
4 ounces	Tomato juice
1/2 small	Apple
	Coffee or tea
	Protein supplement

Twenty-Ninth Day #29 *(continued)*

**EXERCISE AND BRISK WALK—
20 MINUTES COMBINED**
   then

RELAXING BATH "LIME TONIC"

**Cook with 1 tbs. oil

SNACK: 4 ounces chicken (without skin)
   ½ dill pickle

THIRTIETH DAY—#30

BRISK WALK AND HAIR TREATMENT

BREAKFAST

4 ounces	Ground beef patty
4 slices	Cucumber
	Coffee or tea
	Protein supplement

EXERCISE—15 MINUTES AND MANICURE

LUNCH

4 ounces	Turkey (without skin)
2 small	Summer squash**
1 slice	Whole wheat toast (dry)
½ small	Apple
	Coffee or tea
	Protein supplement

**FACIAL "GARDEN OF EDEN" AND PEDICURE
AND SHAMPOO AND SET**

DINNER

5 ounces	Chicken (without skin)
1 cup	Cole slaw
3 ounces	Chow mein
	Coffee or tea
	Protein supplement

BEAUTY RITUAL: LAST NIGHT CELEBRATION:
   1 cocktail—your favorite
   1 special snack—your choice

**Cook with 1 tbs. oil

More Quick Ways to Achieve Lasting Beauty

CHAPTER SIXTEEN

Effective Non-Crash Diet

If you are anxious to "Play the Beauty Game" and have only 10 or 15 pounds to lose, you might like to try this 1200 calorie a day diet for four to six weeks. You can safely and comfortably lose 2 pounds a week on this regimen.

If you have more than 10 or 15 pounds to lose, you can still utilize this diet, but eliminate those foods marked with asterisks. This way, you can lose 3 or 4 pounds per week and speed up the process.

General words of caution: Wherever coffee or tea is listed, you may add lemon and low calorie sugar substitute to tea, and skim milk or non-dairy milk product and sugar substitute to coffee.

Experiment with the various low-calorie salad dressings on the market. Some are more palatable than others. Individual taste will determine which one you'll find easier to live with.

FIRST DAY

BREAKFAST:

    1 orange (in juice form or eaten in sections)
    1 poached egg
    *1 slice toast with 1 pat of butter
    black coffee or tea

LUNCH:

    Chef's Salad Bowl:
        lettuce
        green beans
        asparagus tips
        tomato slices
        4 sardines
        garnish with green pepper strips
        1 cup cottage cheese
        low calorie dressing
      *1 slice bread—½ pat of butter
      *1 apple
      iced coffee or tea

DINNER:

    *1 glass (4 oz.) grape juice
    4 oz. lean hamburger patty
    sliced tomatoes
    1 serving asparagus or brussels sprouts
    *1 slice bread—½ pat of butter
    small mixed green salad with 1 tablespoon low
        calorie dressing
    ¼ slice cantaloupe
    coffee or tea

SECOND DAY

BREAKFAST:

    ½ grapefruit
    1 serving hot oatmeal (with skim milk or
        non-dairy product)
    *1 slice bread—1 pat of butter
    coffee or tea

Second Day (*continued*)

LUNCH:
> 1 cup bouillon
> stuffed tomato with ½ cup cottage cheese
> *1 slice bread—½ pat of butter
> *1 apple
> coffee or tea

DINNER:
> glass of tomato juice (6 oz.)
> minute steak (3 oz.)
> 1 serving green beans
> *1 small ear of corn
> ¼ honeydew melon
> coffee or tea

THIRD DAY

BREAKFAST:
> 1 orange (juice or eaten in sections)
> 1 serving dry cereal with skim milk or non-dairy
>   milk product
> *1 cup strawberries
> *1 slice toast with ½ pat butter
> coffee or tea

LUNCH:
> 1 cup chicken broth (clear)
> shrimp salad:
>   lettuce
>   1 small tomato in wedges
>   6 jumbo shrimp
>   3 stalks celery diced
>   2 strips green pepper
>   low calorie dressing
> *1 slice bread—1 pat butter
> 1 slice fresh pineapple
> coffee or tea

DINNER:
> 4 oz. sliced white meat of turkey (remove skin)
> 1 serving squash
> *1 slice bread and 1 pat butter

Third Day *(continued)*

    lettuce and tomato salad
    low calorie dressing
    1 cup raspberries
    coffee or tea

FOURTH DAY

BREAKFAST:

    ½ grapefruit
    1 soft boiled egg
    *1 slice toast—1 pat butter
    coffee or skim milk

LUNCH:

    1 serving fish (5 oz.)
    *1 serving asparagus with lemon butter (melt 1 pat butter
        and ¼ juice lemon. For lower calorie menu, eliminate
        butter)
    ½ small tomato
    *1 slice bread—1 pat butter
    ¼ serving cantaloupe
    coffee, tea, skim milk

DINNER:

    2 slices smoked salmon on 2 Melba toast rounds
    4 oz. broiled chicken (remove skin)
    1 serving squash
    1 small tomato
    *½ cup strawberries with milk
    coffee or tea

FIFTH DAY

BREAKFAST:

    small orange (eaten in sections)
    1 poached egg
    *1 slice toast—1 pat of butter
    coffee or tea

LUNCH:

    vegetable aspic salad:
        unflavored gelatin

Fifth Day (*continued*)

    1 bouillon cube
    ½ cup tomato juice
    6 asparagus spears
    1 chopped hard boiled egg
    mold, chill, serve
  *1 slice bread—1 pat butter
    1 slice watermelon
    coffee or tea

DINNER:

    4 shrimp on small bed of lettuce
    3½ ozs. lean roast beef
  *1 small baked potato with ½ pat of butter
    1 serving squash
  *1 apple (on low calorie diet substitute ¼ slice cantaloupe)
    coffee or tea

SIXTH DAY

BREAKFAST:

    ½ grapefruit
    1 poached egg
  *1 slice toast—1 pat butter
    coffee or tea

LUNCH:

    4 ozs. broiled chicken (remove skin)
    1 serving broccoli
  *1 small baked potato
    lettuce and tomato salad
    low calorie dressing
  *1 pear
    coffee or tea

DINNER:

    1 cup beef bouillon
    4 oz. filet of sole (topped with lemon juice)
  *1 small ear of corn
    1 serving squash
    ½ tomato sliced
    ¼ slice cantaloupe
    coffee or tea

SEVENTH DAY

BREAKFAST:
    ½ grapefruit
    1 serving oatmeal (with skim milk or non-dairy
       milk product)
    *1 slice toast—1 pat butter
    coffee or tea

LUNCH:
    shrimp salad:
       lettuce
       8 shrimp
       3 stalks celery diced
       1 scallion (optional)
       ½ small tomato
     *1 hard boiled egg
       6 asparagus spears
       low calorie dressing
    *1 slice bread—1 pat butter
    Coffee or tea

DINNER:
    ½ broiled lobster
    *Made with 1 pat of butter; for lower calorie diet,
       use 1 pat diet margarine
    1 serving spinach
    small mixed green salad
    low calorie dressing
    coffee, tea, skim milk
    ½ cantaloupe

"Fad and Fantasy" Diets

CHAPTER SEVENTEEN

"Fad and Fantasy" Diets

The following fad diets are NOT recommended. It is our considered opinion that unless you are not really obese, and have only four to seven pounds to lose—which you can do rapidly on these diets—that you should forget the "It took me 20 years to become a size 44, but I want to be a size 14 tomorrow" routine and concentrate on adjusting to a *lifelong* program of sensible eating. However, there are always those who MUST try everything once . . . so, if your doctor gives you the green light, try a few of these food fad fantasy diets. . . . and good luck!

Grapefruit and Fish Diet

If you do NOT deviate . . . or add anything to the menus below . . . you should drop 5 to 7 pounds within a week.

BREAKFAST:
    ½ grapefruit
    3 ounces of any fish (broiled or baked with lemon juice)
    coffee or tea

LUNCH:

½ grapefruit
4 ounces of any fish (broiled or baked with lemon juice)
¼ wedge lettuce—low cal dressing
2 stalks celery
½ small tomato
coffee or tea

DINNER:

½ grapefruit
4 ounces of any fish (broiled or baked with lemon juice)
1 cup green beans
coffee or tea

SNACK:

Before retiring, ½ grapefruit

"Orange Juice and Iron Will" Diet

One of the newer fad diets currently in vogue is this one. To be fair, we've talked with more than a dozen people who swear by this one. Each of them had lost a minimum of 20 pounds in 5 weeks . . . each also admitted the going was *very rough!*

Again, we cannot emphasize too strongly our own personal prejudice against diets of this type. Ready? Here goes.

For the first four days, you may consume nothing—absolutely nothing—but orange juice or orange slices. Morning, noon, and night that's all you may "indulge" in.

FIFTH DAY

BREAKFAST:

½ grapefruit
3 ounces of chicken
coffee or tea

LUNCH:

  ¼ wedge lettuce
  ½ small tomato
  2 celery stalks
  low-cal dressing
  6 jumbo shrimp
  coffee or tea

DINNER:

  1 cup bouillon
  4 ounces broiled chicken (skinless)
  1 cup green beans
  coffee or tea

The menus are the same for the 6th and 7th days. All you can vary is the luncheon meal. You may substitute 4 ounces of any fish for the shrimp. The same rules regarding the artificial sweetening of coffee and tea apply here. Also you may include low-cal carbonated beverages as previously mentioned.

Repeat this routine for seven days, varying your selection of fish to suit your own palate.

Nothing else may be consumed during the day with the exception of a low calorie artifically sweetened carbonated soft drink, which you may have as you desire. Also, you may add a low-cal sweetener to your coffee and tea, plus a lemon wedge in your tea. EVERYTHING ELSE IS VERBOTEN!

Variation

Instead of chicken, you may substitute the equivalent amount of fish broiled with lemon for the 5th, 6th and 7th days. The remainder of the diet is the same.

Weight Stabilizing Recipes

Once you've reached your desired weight, don't play tug-of-war with the scales. But if you *do* find yourself regaining a few pounds, *take them off immediately.*

Beginning on the next page you will find some recipes for main dishes, salads, vegetables and desserts that are tasty, low calorie dishes. They will help you to maintain your correct weight.

Incidentally, here are a few more general dietary hints: Grapefruit can be a dieter's friend. It's loaded with Vitamin C, which helps prevent respiratory infections and is important in the maintenance of strong teeth and bones. If utilized in various forms, the grapefruit can be a marvelous weapon in your tug-of-war against fattening foods!

To help curb your appetite, any one of the following food combinations consumed 1/2 hour before a meal is very effective:

145

2 Melba toast rounds
        and
½ cup tomato juice

1 cup black coffee or tea
2 stalks of celery stuffed with cottage cheese

1 dill pickle
½ of a small fresh tomato

SUPER CHEF'S SALAD

250 calories per serving

⅓ head lettuce
3 stalks celery—diced
1 tomato sliced
pinch of salt
2 ounces white meat chicken (skinless)
1 scallion—cut up fine (optional)
6 shrimp
dash of pepper
1½ tablespoon "Good Life" French dressing (or any low calorie dressing)

Break lettuce and place in bottom of bowl. Add celery and onions. Pour dressing over lettuce and celery. Toss. Add tomatoes, chicken and shrimp. Season and serve.

CHECKERBOARD

8 servings
1 serving (½ cup) 50 calories

1 envelope low-cal vanilla pudding
1 envelope low-cal chocolate pudding
4 cups skim (low-fat) milk

Empty vanilla pudding into pan. Add 1 cup of milk. Stir mixture well. Add 1 more cup of milk. Cook mixture until it comes to a boil. Cool 10 minutes. Stir. Chill until set.

Repeat directions with chocolate pudding. When both mixtures are well chilled remove from refrigerator and separately whip each mixture until it is creamy. Then take tall sherbet glasses and alternately spoon layers of vanilla and chocolate puddings into glass.

SLIM DIP MIX

5 servings
75 calories each

> 1 8 oz. can minced clams
> ¼ cup skim milk
> 12 ounces—hoop or pot cheese
> ½ teaspoon onion salt
> 1 teaspoon Worcestershire Sauce
> celery stalks
> carrot sticks

Drain liquid from clams and pour into a bowl. Then blend in cheese, milk, onion salt and sauce. Be sure the ingredients are very well mixed (use an electric blender if you can).

Next, add clams. Chill for an hour or two. To serve—place on each salad bowl ¼ cup clam dip. Arrange celery and carrots around it—then dig in!

RADIANT RADISH SALAD

6 servings
29 calories each

> 2 bunches radishes, washed and trimmed
> 2 tablespoons sour cream
> 2 tablespoons low-cal mayonnaise
> 1 tablespoon skim milk
> pinch of pepper
> ½ teaspoon salt
> lettuce

Chop radishes up in thin slivers and place in a bowl. Stir in sour cream, milk, mayonnaise and seasonings. Place in refrigerator for ½ hour, or until ready to serve.

Arrange salad plates with a portion of lettuce, then top with radish mixture.

LEMON SNOW

5 servings
1 serving 50 calories

>   1 envelope low-cal vanilla pudding
>   1 cup lemon juice
>   ½ envelope low-cal lemon gelatin
>   pinch of salt
>   ½ cup boiling water
>   2 egg whites
>   1 thin slice of fresh lemon

Place pudding in pan. Add ¼ cup lemon juice. Stir until well mixed. Add remaining juice. Cook until mixture comes to a boil. Remove from heat. Dissolve lemon gelatin and pinch of salt in boiling water. Combine with pudding mixture and chill until it thickens. Pour into empty ice tray. Freeze until mixture is thick in the center. Place mixture in a well chilled bowl. Beat until smooth. Then beat egg whites until they are stiff. Fold into mixture. Return to ice tray and freeze until firm. Stir occasionally.

Before serving, allow mixture to stand at room temperature for 10 minutes. Garnish with thin lemon wedges.

PINEAPPLE BROILED CHICKEN

4 servings (¼ chicken per serving)
150 calories per serving

Place cleaned, washed broiler (or fryer) chicken halves skin down in lined broiler pan. Squeeze pinch of fresh lemon over chicken. Dot with diet margarine. Season with small amount of pepper and salt substitute. Place chicken at least 5 inches from flames. Turn broiler to 375 degrees. Broil 15 to 20 minutes. Turn. Squeeze more lemon on top. Broil 20 minutes or until chicken is nicely browned. About 10 minutes before chicken is done add 2 slices of diet pineapple to each chicken half.

TUNA-POTATO SALAD

6 servings
1 serving (1 cup) 95 calories

>   1 head lettuce
>   2½ cups potatoes, cooked and diced

2 cups water-packed tuna
2 hard-boiled eggs
4 stalks celery—diced
2 scallions—diced (optional)
2 strips green pepper—diced
dash of pepper
pinch of salt
dash of paprika
low-calorie dressing—1 tablespoon on each serving

For each serving place a portion of lettuce at bottom of bowl. Add some green peppers, onions and celery. Add a cup of mixed tuna, potatoes and eggs in center. Season each bowl individually and top with low-cal dressing.

BAKED ZUCCHINI

4 servings
35 calories per serving (1 squash)

4 zucchini (small)
1 chopped onion
1 tablespoon diet margarine
pinch of salt and pepper
1 tablespoon bread crumbs

Wash zucchini and cut off ends. Boil squash until tender (about 12-15 minutes). Remove from water. Cut from top of squash 1 thin slice and place in mixing bowl. Gently scoop out inside of squash and add to bowl. Mix in onion and seasoning. Replace mixture in square shells. Sprinkle on bread crumbs. Place in broiler for 20 minutes at 400 degrees.

BROWNIES

65 calories each

Buy a prepared angel food cake mix and follow package directions.
Before pouring batter in thin sheets in baking pan add one small jar (6 ounces) of low calorie chocolate sauce, plus 1 cup walnuts. Bake. Yield: 3 dozen brownies.

NOTE: If you have a great deal to lose, resist the temptation to bake these!

HEAVENLY CRISPS

11 calories each (small piece)

> ⅓ cup miniature marshmallows
> 1 cup Rice Crispies

Put both ingredients in a non-stick skillet. Stir over a low-medium flame until marshmallows begin to melt and Rice Crispies are well blended. Pour onto a sheet of aluminum foil. Cool. Break off small pieces and eat.

LOW-CAL ESPRESSO PUDDING

8 servings
1 serving (½ cup) 50 calories

> 1 envelope low-cal chocolate pudding
> 1 cup brewed espresso coffee
> 1 cup cold water
> low-cal whipped cream topping

Put pudding in pan. Add ½ cup water. Mix thoroughly. Add remaining water and coffee. Cook until mixture comes to a boil. Remove from heat and spoon into serving cup. Chill. vBefore serving, top with 1 squirt low-cal whipped cream.

TOMATO BOUILLON

2 servings
28 calories per cup

> 1½ cups tomato juice
> 1 stalk celery diced
> 1 slice of onion
> ½ teaspoon pepper

Combine ingredients in pan. Heat just to gentle boil. Allow to simmer for 8 minutes. Strain. Reheat and serve. Garnish with a thin slice of lemon.

LOW CALORIE—MELLOW YELLOW SALAD

4 servings
1 mold (22 calories)

> 1 envelope yellow D-Zerta (low-cal) gelatin

⅔ cup raw carrots—grated
¼ cup diet pineapple
2 cups boiling water
1 pinch salt
1 tablespoon vinegar

Dissolve gelatin and salt in boiling water. Add vinegar. Chill until partially thick. Add carrots and pineapple. Pour into individual molds. Chill. Serve on a bed of lettuce.

BROILED TOMATOES AND CHICKEN LIVERS

2 servings
85 calories each

    6 chicken livers
    2 tomatoes
    ½ teaspoon polyunsaturated diet margarine
    pinch of salt
    1 teaspoon flour

After livers are washed, sprinkle on pinch of salt. Dip each liver in thin flour batter. Wash and slice tomatoes. Add margarine. Place in shallow pan and broil at 375 until livers are browned.

GRAPEFRUIT SALAD

4 servings
200 calories per serving

    2 cups water-packed tuna, or skinless chicken chunks
    salad greens
    2 cups grapefruit sections
    4 radishes
    1 cucumber, sliced

Arrange salad greens on a serving plate or individual bowl. Place tuna or chicken in the middle. Surround with cucumber slices, top with grapefruit sections, garnish with radish slices.

GRAPEFRUIT SALAD DRESSING

Makes 1¼ cups
20 calories per tablespoon

¼ cup catsup
2 tablespoons polyunsaturated salad oil
1 cup grapefruit juice
½ teaspoon dry mustard
½ teaspoon paprika
⅛ teaspoon pepper
½ teaspoon salt (salt substitute)
1 teaspoon sugar
2 teaspoons cornstarch

Combine dry ingredients in saucepan. Stir in grapefruit juice. Place over medium heat and bring to a boil, stirring constantly. Boil one minute. Remove from heat. Stir in remaining ingredients. Chill. Stir before serving.

FRESH MELON BOWL

6 servings
½ cup serving (25 calories)

1 cup Honeydew melon balls
¼ cup strawberries
1 cup cantaloupe balls
1 cup Crenshaw melon balls
½ tablespoon lemon juice

Combine melon balls and strawberries. Squeeze lemon juice on top. Chill.

BROILED HALIBUT

3 servings
165 calories per serving (⅓ pound)

1 lb. halibut (filets)
½ tablespoon diet margarine
1 tablespoon lemon juice
pinch of salt
dash of pepper
sprinkle of paprika (optional)

Turn oven to 375. Arrange fish on lined broiler pan. Brush with margarine, add lemon juice, salt, pepper and paprika. Broil for 12 minutes, 3" from flames, or until fish is easy to flake with a fork. Do not turn. Fish is done when cooked in this manner on one side.

CHOCOLATE SUPREME

7 servings
1 serving (½ cup—45 calories)

 1 envelope low-cal chocolate pudding
 2 cups skim (low-fat) milk
 2 egg whites
 2 tablespoons sugar (or substitute)

Place pudding in saucepan. Add ¼ cup of milk. Stir until mixed. Blend in rest of milk. Cook until mixture comes to a gentle boil, stirring occasionally. Remove pan from heat. Beat egg whites until stiff. Add sugar to egg whites. Beat until mixture peaks. Stir pudding into egg whites. Blend well. Spoon into individual cups. Chill until firm.

DIETER'S DELIGHT OMELET

1 serving
160 calories

 1 egg
 1 tablespoon water
 pinch of salt
 ¼ cup diced green pepper
 ¼ cup diced onion (optional)
 ¼ cup sliced tomatoes
 2 sliced mushrooms (fresh)
 1½ tablespoons diet margarine

Break egg. Beat. Add water until egg white and yolk are well blended. Add other ingredients except margarine.
In a skillet, slowly melt margarine. Pour in egg mixture. Watch constantly and tip pan to get all uncooked portions of omelet done. When this occurs, use fork or spatula to roll one corner of omelet over the other.

Here are a few alternates to the "Good Life" French dressing mentioned elsewhere. The first one contains only 10 calories per tablespoon. The second and third dressings have 15 calories per tablespoon.

FLAVORFUL FRENCH DRESSING

Yield 1⅓ cups

   ½ cup water
   1 tablespoon cornstarch
   1 cup canned tomato juice
   2 tablespoons salad oil
   ¼ cup vinegar
   1 teaspoon salt
   ¼ teaspoon prepared horse-radish
   ¼ teaspoon paprika
   ¼ teaspoon onion salt
   ½ teaspoon Worcestershire
   ¼ teaspoon celery salt
   scant ⅛ teaspoon dry mustard
   2 dashes garlic salt

Day before serving:

(1) In a small saucepan, stir water into cornstarch until blended; add tomato juice; stir constantly over low heat until slightly thickened.

(2) Remove from heat; cool; add salad oil, vinegar, salt, horse-radish, paprika, onion salt, Worcestershire, celery salt, mustard and garlic salt; beat with hand beater or electric mixer until smooth and well blended.

(3) Store, covered, in refrigerator. Use as needed, shaking well before serving.

COTTAGE CHEESE—DILL DRESSING

Yield 1½ cups

   1 cup creamed cottage cheese
   ½ teaspoon salt
   ⅛ teaspoon cayenne pepper
   ¼ cup sour cream
   2 tablespoons water
   ¼ cup fresh dill, finely snipped

In a blender jar, mix cottage cheese, salt, pepper, sour cream and water. Blend until very smooth. Transfer to a clean glass jar. Stir in dill. Cover. Refrigerate several hours before using.

GLEAMING GODDESS DRESSING

Yield 1½ cups

1 clove garlic
½ teaspoon salt
½ teaspoon dry mustard
1 teaspoon Worcestershire
2 tablespoons anchovy paste
2 tablespoons tarragon-wine vinegar
3 tablespoons snipped chives
⅓ cup snipped parsley
⅛ teaspoon black pepper
1 cup boiled salad dressing (Use dressing above)

Day before serving:

(1) In a small bowl, crush garlic through a garlic press and mix with salt, or crush garlic and salt together with back of spoon.

(2) Add mustard, Worcestershire, anchovy paste, vinegar, chives, parsley and pepper; stir until smooth. Stir in boiled salad dressing until smooth.

(3) Cover tightly; refrigerate overnight. Use as a topping for salads—Goddess Shrimp Salad or as a dressing for any salad greens.

SUCCULENT SALMON SLIMMER

3 servings
1 serving— (4 ounces) 255 calories

2 pounds Salmon steaks
½ teaspoon salt
¼ teaspoon white pepper
4 ounces fresh or canned sliced mushrooms
½ cup sliced scallions (optional)
2 tablespoons diet margarine

Place fish in baking dish. Sprinkle with salt and pepper. Combine remaining ingredients and spread over top of dish. Bake in moderate oven 350 degrees for 25 to 30 minutes or until fish flakes easily with a fork.

SOLE FOR THE SOUL

6 servings
132 calories per serving

        1 can (about 7 ounces) crab meat, drained
        ½ teaspoon dry mustard
        ¼ teaspoon leaf marjoram, crumbled
        ¼ teaspoon Worcestershire sauce
        6 fresh filets of sole (about 1½ pounds)
        6 peppercorns
        4 bay leaves
        1 teaspoon salt
        1 tablespoon lemon juice
        1 cup water
        1 tablespoon flour
        1 tablespoon bottled catsup
        1 teaspoon non-dairy coffee "cream" powder

Break crab meat into small chunks; remove any bony tissue. Place in a small bowl; mix in mustard, marjoram, and Worcestershire sauce. Cut sole filets in half lengthwise. Spoon 2 teaspoonfuls crab mixture on wide end of each piece; roll up, jelly-roll fashion; fasten with wooden picks. Stand rolls on end in a large baking dish. Add peppercorns, bay leaves, salt, lemon juice, and water to baking dish; cover. Bake in slow oven (325°) 30 min. or until fish flakes easily. Lift fish rolls carefully from liquid with a pancake turner to a platter; keep hot while making sauce.
Strain liquid from fish into a bowl, then measure 1 cupful into a small saucepan; discard remainder. Stir flour, catsup, and powdered "cream" into saucepan; cook, stirring constantly, until sauce thickens slightly and boils 1 minute. Place 2 fish rolls on each of 6 heated serving plates; spoon about 1 tablespoon of sauce over each.

PARMESAN TOMATOES
(2 halves)

Each serving 50 calories

        2 tomatoes
        1 tablespoon chopped parsley
        ½ tablespoon diet margarine
        1 tablespoon Parmesan cheese
        dash of salt and pepper

For each serving, slice one tomato in half. Place on a shallow broiler pan. Season. Sprinkle cheese on top. Add margarine. Broil for five minutes in 350° oven.

TASTY BRUSSELS SPROUTS

4 servings, each serving 1 cup—50 calories

> 1 pound brussel sprouts
> 1 tablespoon diet margarine
> 1 cup mushrooms (water-packed)
> dash of pepper and salt

Cook sprouts until tender. Drain. Add margarine and mushrooms. Heat until margarine melts and mushrooms are hot. Serve immediately.

ITALIAN CAULIFLOWER

4 servings
1 serving (1/4 head) 43 calories

> 2 tablespoons diet margarine
> 2 tablespoons Parmesan cheese

Cook cauliflower until tender. Drain. Melt margarine in a saucepan. Add cheese. Spoon this over cauliflower and serve immediately.

FILET OF SOLE

6 servings
150 calories per serving

> 2 pounds sole filets
> 1/4 cup chopped onion
> 2 cups sliced mushrooms (fresh or canned)
> 2 tablespoons polyunsaturated margarine
> 2 tablespoons lemon juice
> 1/4 teaspoon pepper
> 1 teaspoon oregano

In a large skillet sauté mushrooms and onions in margarine until tender. Place sole in pan. Sprinkle remaining ingredients over fish. Cover. Simmer for 20 minutes.

MILADY'S SEAFOOD SALAD

200 calories per serving

> 1/3 head lettuce
> 2 stalks celery—diced

    2 strips green pepper—diced
    1 scallion—chopped finely (optional)
    1 tomato—quartered
    8 jumbo shrimp
    2 small lobster tails
    2 tablespoons low calorie dressing

Break lettuce and put in a bowl. Add celery, green pepper and onions. Spoon 1½ tablespoons of dressing over dish. Add cooked shrimp and lobster tails. Add tomato wedges. Use remaining dressing. Season with a dash of pepper.

BEANS, MUSHROOMS SUPREME

3 servings
1 serving (1 cup) —35 calories

    Green beans—1 package frozen
    ½ cup mushrooms (canned in water)
    Dash of salt & pepper
    1 tablespoon diet margarine

Cook beans as per package directions. Season. In a separate pan heat mushrooms in water. Drain and add to beans. Serve immediately.

BAYOU SHRIMP FEAST

6 servings—200 calories each

    3 onions—peeled and sliced thin
    1 small can (4 ounces) chopped mushrooms
    ½ cup diced green pepper
    ½ teaspoon salt
    ¼ teaspoon curry powder
    pinch of paprika
    ⅛ teaspoon pepper
    1 can (12 ounces) stewed tomatoes
    2 teaspoons (or equivalent) low-cal sweetener
    1 pound cleaned shrimp
    3 cups noodles (cooked)

Combine onions, mushrooms and liquid, green pepper, all seasonings and tomatoes in a large frying pan. Stir in low-cal sweetener. Heat slowly. Stir constantly. When mixture reaches boiling point, simmer for 12 min. (until onions and green peppers are tender). Next, add shrimp. Simmer for 10 more minutes until shrimp are well heated. For each serving, spoon a portion of hot noodles on to your dinner plate. Top with shrimp mixture.

HONG KONG CHICKEN AND VEGETABLES

3 servings—275 calories each

> 2 boneless, skinless chicken breasts (8 ounces each)
> 5 ounces French-style frozen green beans
> ½ teaspoon salt
> ½ cup celery—diced
> ½ pound bean sprouts (drained)
> ⅛ teaspoon pepper
> 1 tablespoon cornstarch
> 1½ tablespoons soy sauce
> 1½ tablespoons cider vinegar
> 1½ cups cooked rice
> 1 tomato (cut in wedges)

Cut chicken breasts into strips about ½" wide. Sprinkle salt in a frying pan. Add chicken. Sauté for 10 min. stirring frequently. Push to one side. Place frozen beans in frying pan. Cook for 5 min. separating beans as they thaw. Stir in celery, ½ cup water, bean sprouts, vinegar and pepper. Heat to boiling point. Cover. Simmer for 5 more minutes. Put cornstarch and 1 tablespoon of water in a cup. Blend. Stir in soy sauce. Add to mixture in frying pan. Cook until entire mixture thickens and boils—about 4 minutes. Stir constantly.
Place tomato wedges on top. Cover. Steam for 5 minutes. To serve, spoon a portion of hot, cooked rice on each plate. In the center place a portion of your Hong Kong Chicken. Serve immediately. This dish is really quite divine for dieters!

Part V

Life Is a Battle—Win It!

Courage is the first of human qualities because it is the quality which guarantees all the others.

—WINSTON CHURCHILL

Exercises—American Style

If you are one of those women with a slender waistline, well-shaped legs and shoulders, and a lovely bust, then the perfection of your figure can be thrown out of harmony if your hips are too large. If this be your case, your problem is one of slenderizing the hips without disturbing the perfection of the rest of your figure. The hips are particularly subject to fatty deposits and the only sure solution is in exercising. Perhaps you have already tried this method of slenderizing your hips without success, but the solution *is* there. The fault may have been in your way of practicing the exercises, or in the exercises themselves. If you follow an established exercise plan daily, it will do more to aid your particular case than will expending energy in haphazard exercising. Your program must be arranged so that the hip region is the most exercised.

Begin today to devote the prescribed time to the movements described. On the first few days, do only

163

three of the movements. When you have mastered these, then every two days learn how to do another of the exercises. Eventually you will be able to do all of these movements in the time allotted for daily exercise. The more quickly and thoroughly you do each movement, the more value you gain from it. The movements should be done rhythmically and forcefully, with all effort concentrated on the hip region. Proper exercise, proper diet, proper attitude—these are the three essentials which will help you to achieve lasting beauty.

"Face Facts Fast"

Throw your head as far back as possible; while in this position swiftly open and close lips in a popping motion one dozen times. Turn head to the left, look upward over shoulder, repeat mouth exercise. Do the same with head looking over right shoulder.

"One Dozen Poses"

With arms hanging straight down at sides, lift both shoulders up as high as possible, then drop them down to normal position. Up. Down. Up. Down. Repeat, one dozen times. Then lift elbows at sides to bust level, press fingertips together in front of bust. Swing elbows behind you as if trying to make them meet in back. Return to front position, touching fingertips. Repeat one dozen times.

"Hip, Hip, Away!"

Balance yourself on the edge of a straight chair. Tip

the buttocks forward and knees flexed, extend legs forward as far as you can. Point your toes.

Place hands at sides of the pelvic joint, elbows wide, and keep them there throughout the exercise.

Keep ribs high, back straight, head in line with the spine, bend the torso forward as far as you can.

Slowly return to erect sitting position.

Leg and Ankle Shaper

Sit on the edge of a straight chair. Head held high, back straight.

Tip buttocks forward and rest hands lightly on thighs, just above the knees.

With knees together and slightly flexed, extend the legs forward as far as you can and point the toes.

Cross the left foot over the right ankle, extending the left leg and pointing the left foot as much as possible. Feel the stretch and pull from the lower back through the buttocks, thigh, calf, and foot.

Uncross the feet and then cross the right foot over the left ankle.

Repeat four times slowly. Goal: Work up to fifteen times.

For Slimmer Ankles and Shapely Knees

Stand tall, place one hand on the back of a straight chair.

Rise up on the flat of your toes.

With knees pressed together, tip the buttocks forward and bend deeply at the knees.

Now, without moving the hips, slowly turn the knees to the right, then to the left.

Begin slowly—repeat four times. Goal: Fifteen times.

"Arms Race"—#1

Stand with one foot 6″ in front of the other. Slowly rise up on the flat of your toes.

Raise both arms above your head, keep shoulders down, elbows flexed, hands and fingers pointed straight up, palms facing each other.

Hold this position, walk slowly forward on the flat of the toes. Take twelve steps . . . pause . . . repeat.

"Arms Race"—#2

Raise elbows to shoulder level with forearm hanging in a straight line from the elbow, and fingers pointed forward. Swing arms out to the side like a pendulum twelve times. (Be sure to keep elbows at shoulder height.)

For Firm Thighs and a Slim Waist

Stand erect, legs spread about 18″ apart.

Place the side of the hands at the pelvic joint, thumbs back and fingers forward.

Shift weight to left foot and then bend the upper torso to the left, keeping the ribs up and shoulders down and keeping a long straight line along the right side of the body from the torso to the toes.

Shift back to the first position and then to the right.

Start by doing this five times in succession. Goal: fifteen times.

To Slim Hips and Thighs

Balance yourself on the edge of a straight chair. Tip the buttocks forward and, with knees flexed, extend the legs forward as far as you can and point the toes.

Place the hands at the sides of the pelvic joint, with elbows wide, and keep them there throughout the exercise.

Keeping the ribs high, back straight, and head in line with the spine, bend the torso forward as far as you can.

Slowly return to erect sitting position.

Start out doing this five times. Goal: fifteen times.

To Slim the Waistline

A. Stand with feet wide apart and arms stretched straight out at sides. Twist body as far as possible first to left then to right turning only upper part of body and stretching from the waist.

B. Stand with feet wide apart and arms stretched out at sides. Lean to right, keeping arms straight, so right arm reaches as close as possible to floor. Then lean to left, reaching left arm toward floor as far as possible. Six times on each side.

Goal: Work up to ten times on each side.

To Correct That Roll of Fat at the Back of Waistline

Holding knees stiff, raise one leg off floor as high as possible. (Actually you are raising hip.) Repeat first with right foot then with left, keeping knees stiff, and walk across floor in this goosestep manner.

For Knees and Inner Thighs

Stand with feet wide apart, hands on hips. Pull in diaphragm, tuck in derrière, keeping back straight. Bend knees slowly. Go down in a slow deep bend and return to standing position. Try bending a little deeper each day. (When doing housework during the day, instead of bending over to dust, open and close drawers, etc., bend at the knees instead, always keeping back straight.) Six knee bends to start.

Goal: An even dozen per day.

"Mata Hari's Revenge"

For lovely legs and ankles sit on the edge of a straight chair with head held high, back straight.

Tip buttocks forward and rest hands lightly on thighs, just above the knees. Knees together and slightly flexed, extend legs forward as far as you can. Point your toes. Cross the left foot over the right ankle, extending the left leg and pointing the left foot as much as possible. Feel the stretch and pull from the lower back through the buttocks, thigh, calf, and foot. Uncross the feet and then cross the right foot over the left ankle.

Then stand tall, place one hand on the back of a straight chair. Rise up on the flat of your toes.

With knees pressed together, tip your buttocks forward and bend deeply at the knees. Now, without moving your hips, slowly turn the knees to the right, then to the left.

Do these at least ten minutes a day and you'll have legs fit for a delectable "spy."

To Firm the Muscles of Your Neck and Face

Throw head as far back as possible; while in this position rapidly open and close lips in a popping motion, fifteen times. Turn head to the left and looking upward over shoulder, repeat mouth exercise. Do the same with head looking over right shoulder.

To Eliminate Shoulder Fat

A. With arms hanging straight down at sides, lift both shoulders up as high as possible, then drop them down to normal position. Up. Down. Up. Down. Repeat fifteen times.

B. Lift elbows out at sides to bust level, and press fingertips together in front of bust. Then swing elbows back as if trying to make them meet in back. Return to front position, touching fingertips. Repeat twelve times.

To Firm Muscles of Abdomen and Diaphragm

Pull diaphragm in as far as possible to 1-2-3 count. Hold for a few seconds then push diaphragm out. Repeat twelve times, night and morning.

Thigh Toner

Use a leather belt you have around the house as a prop for this exercise. Place weight on right foot, bend left knee slightly. Place belt just below the knee and grasp firmly. At this point, your shoulders should be erect. Now slowly begin to straighten spine as you elevate the knee. Change legs. Try 3 times with each knee bent. Increase to 5 . . . then 10 . . . watch thighs tighten.

With the arrival of minis and micro-minis, beauty from the waist down is more important than ever.

Not only your legs, but also your hips are being exposed to more air and eye so girdle and corset tricks by themselves just won't do the proper job today.

Usually if there is an excess of body weight it will be localized in the hips, thighs and buttocks. These regions are particularly susceptible to fat accumulations because of the increased infiltration of liquid and fat into the tissues.

Waist

Corsets and girdles can disguise a figure to give the appearance of a trim waistline and a flat stomach. However, it is much better to have firm retaining muscles which hold the organs in place at all times rather than to depend upon a foundation garment to do the entire job.

A. Stand erect with your feet together. Stretch your arms overhead and clasp your hands together. B-e-n-d away as far as possible, keeping your arms straight as you move them quickly in small circles from front to back. Pulling upward from the hip muscles, b-e-n-d as far as possible to the other side as you continue the circles. Repeat five times. It is very important to pull.

Hips, Thighs, Buttocks

Heavy thighs and fat buttocks are way "out" for today's "in" look. One excellent means for remodeling the body form is manual massage. The concentrated effects of massages are particularly helpful in reducing fat and water accumulations in the cells as well as helping to make the muscles more supple and stimulating the circulation. For massaging at home, the roller or ball type body massagers, used with a slenderizing cream, are excellent.

A. FIFTEEN-SECOND TENSER is a good exercise for strengthening buttock muscles. Simply tense those muscles, hold for fifteen seconds, then let go. Repeat five times.

B. Lie down on your back with your feet and legs flat on the floor. Raise your arms over your head. S-l-o-w-l-y raise the top of your body forward until you are sitting. Keep legs and feet flat on the floor. Now, as slowly as possible, lower yourself back to your original position.

If you already have a slender waistline, well-shaped legs and shoulders, and a lovely bosom, but the harmony of your figure is disturbed because your hips are too large, your problem is special. *You must slenderize your hips*—which are particularly subject to fattening —without disturbing the perfection of the rest of your figure.

"Don't Thigh—Waist A-Weigh!"

Stand erect, legs spread fifteen inches apart.

Place the side of the hands at the pelvic joint, thumbs back, fingers forward.

Shift weight to left foot, bend upper torso to the left, keeping ribs up and shoulders down and keeping a long straight line along the right side of the body from the torso to the toes.

Shift back to the original position and then go to the right.

Thigh Slimmer

Lie flat on the floor with your arms spread-eagled, your legs straight. Keeping your knee straight, raise your right leg until it is at a right angle to your body. Then throw your leg across your body and try to touch your left hand with your right toes. Don't lift your shoulders from the floor—only your right leg and hip should move—and don't worry if your toes and hand don't meet. It's trying that counts. Finally, swing your leg to the right, around, up again, and again across to reach for your fingers. Begin with five swings and then switch to the other leg. Work up to twenty go-rounds for each leg.

To Eliminate a Protruding Stomach

Here's an exercise that usually works when all else fails. Lie flat on your back on the floor (on a pad, if you will, but not on a bed) with your knees bent and touching and your feet flat and toed in, about two feet apart and about a foot from your buttocks. Fold your arms over your chest and let yourself "sink into" the floor until every inch of your back, including the small part, is touching the floor. This relaxing process may take as long as five minutes. Then place your arms on the floor beside your body, palms down, and slowly slide your legs down on the floor, feet and knees together. Make a special effort not to arch your back. Now press down with the palms of your hands and slowly raise your legs from the floor, toes pointed, knees straight, back flat on the floor. When you have raised your legs about two feet from the floor, pause and bob them up and down, without touching the floor, five times. *Slowly* lower your legs to the floor, keeping your back flat. Repeat. Note: At first you may have to do one leg at a time, but after a few weeks you should work up to twenty times a day. Allow about two months for signs of flattening.

For Arms and Legs

Stand with one foot 6" in front of the other.

Slowly rise up on the flat of your toes.

Raise both arms above your head, keeping the shoulders down, elbows flexed, and the hands and fingers pointed straight up, palms facing each other.

Holding this position, walk slowly forward on the flat of the toes.

Take twelve steps. Rest. Take twelve more steps. Goal: Work up to sixteen.

To Firm Upper Arms

Raise elbows to shoulder level with forearm hanging in a straight line from the elbow, and fingers pointed forward. Swing arms out to the side like a pendulum twelve times. (Be sure to keep elbows at shoulder height.)

"Slim Gym Waist-Aide"

Stand with feet wide apart, arms stretched straight out at sides. Twist body as far as possible first to left then to right (turning only upper part of body and stretching from the waist). Then stand with feet wide apart and arms stretched out at sides. Lean to right, keeping arms straight, so right arm reaches as close as possible to floor. Then lean to left, reaching left arm toward floor as far as possible. Try at least six times on each side.

"No More Fat-Roll Blues"

Hold your knees stiff. Raise one leg off the floor as high as possible. (Actually you are raising hip.) Repeat first with right foot, then with left. Keep knees stiff. Walk across floor in this goose-step manner. Try five minutes of this a day.

"No More Sad Knees for Me"

Stand with feet wide apart. Place hands on hips. Pull in diaphragm. Tuck in derrière. Keep back straight.

Bend knees slowly. Go down in a slow deep bend. Return to standing position. Try to bend a little deeper with each passing day.

The solution? Just one: Exercise. Believe me, exercise DOES work if done correctly. Don't exercise haphazardly. Follow an established daily plan, one which will do more to aid your cause than harm it.

Yoga and You

In order to achieve lasting beauty, you must have both desire and discipline. Yoga exercises can be aids to physical enhancement and proper body maintenance. As with all things which are written for a mass audience, but which must be INDIVIDUALLY applied, these exercises are for you to take and use if they will make you feel and look better personally. Only you can know your own capacity for physical exercise. Let wise judgment and your desire for a trim shape guide you in their use. Incidentally, in most towns and cities there are professional yoga instructors to consult for more details and for personal supervision, if you wish.

One note of caution: *These exercises must be repeated in the sequence given here.* Never repeat the same posture twice in a row. Respect the method of yoga breathing. ALWAYS observe the rest period between each yoga movement. These general rules are a must because of the basic principles behind these exercises.

Each yoga posture, when correctly executed, controls and exercises only specific muscles while the rest of the body is decontracted. For each posture there is a special way to breathe and, during each rest period, another form of breathing is performed to purify the body of toxins. By following the proper sequence of postures, and observing the rest periods in between, you are making the most efficacious use of yoga. (These are best done on any floor surface.)

1. Face down on the floor, clasp your ankles with your hands in preparation for forming a body arch. Raise your legs and your head while *inhaling*. Hold the position as long as you can *without* exhaling.

NOTE: Spread your legs apart at the beginning of your yoga efforts so as not to make your body ache. Once you are used to this, there will be no concern on that score. At the end of your arch position, release your legs and turn over with your back to the floor and rest.

2. Relaxation: Stretched out on the floor, breathe slowly —*very slowly*—and distend (inflate) the stomach. Take at least two dozen breaths while doing this.

3. Still on your back, draw your knee up toward your face as you exhale. Hold the position for a few moments (be sure your back is flat on the floor with only the head elevated). Change legs while inhaling. Repeat the exercise with each leg, four times altogether.

4. Relaxation—#2.

5. Lying on your back, face looking toward the ceiling, elevate your midriff as high as possible with the aid of your hands; legs held together, heels and shoulders firmly posed. Breathe deeply, expanding the stomach with each breath. Hold this position as long as possible, then ease your midriff to the floor slowly. Do this exercise twice.

6. Relaxation—#2.

7. Seated back on your heels, exhale slowly while bending your head towards the floor and without altering your seated position. Hold this posture as long as you can *without* taking another breath. NOTE: You might find yourself getting a little light headed at first until you learn to exercise the proper body control. Do this only two or three times until it becomes second nature to you—and it WILL.

8. Relaxation—#2.

9. Lying on the floor, stretch out while inhaling and then bend your body towards your legs while exhaling. Rest with your lungs emptied for as long as possible. Keep your stomach held firmly to your legs even if this means bending your knees to do so.

10. Relaxation—#2.

11. Seat yourself on the calf of one leg and place your other foot in front of the knee of the leg on which you are seated. Pose your stomach against the leg while pivoting the shoulders. The movement of your arms may be difficult to control at first. Try to keep them relaxed and it will come easier to you. Pause a moment. Repeat exercise seated on the opposite leg.

12. Relaxation—#2.

13. Stretch out on the floor with your legs interlocked, tailor fashion (legs bent up toward the center of your body) ; rest your arms across the top of your head. Use caution so as not to strain yourself and begin relaxing slowly . . . let your mind drain of all thoughts . . . begin relaxing from the top of your head down . . . think of nothing . . . Remain this way for as long as you are able.

14. Return to relaxation exercise #2.

These fundamental yoga positions will give you a new lease on life if you learn to do them properly and then DO them as your daily act of living.

Spice Up Your Life

If you have decided to go on a reducing diet, there is one item to be considered—a very important item— YOUR MAN. Assuming you are married, or seeing someone on a steady basis, there is no sense gaining a new you and losing the old him! As always "Playing the Beauty Game" *does* require some thought on your part.

Many a newly-trimmed-down *femme* has devoted so much time, energy and effort to reducing that, in the process, she has driven out the man—or men—in her life. Although our diets and beauty rituals are geared toward making you happy and calm while reducing, you WILL still have to be following a rather set routine. What more devotion and love can you show a man than to keep HIS happiness in mind while you are trying to improve yours?

Therefore, while you are sticking to your own diet, unless your hubby or beau prefers going on the diet with you, here are some recipes and tips for cooking *for him* that are guaranteed to make him happy, too.

You will note that, for the most part, these recipes call for the SAME kinds of food as can be found on

178

several of your diets—with one exception—they ARE NOT dietetically oriented. For instance, while you are eating your own chicken—*sans skin*—why not cook him Coq au Vin—chicken in wine. You can put *your* portion in the oven at the same time, eliminating any fattening additives that are suggested.

Catch on? This ability to think of him while helping yourself is an unbeatable combination. Remember you CAN spice up your life just by being considerate and nice. Try it!—You have everything to gain while at the same time you are losing WEIGHT. Each time you "Play the Beauty Game" properly, you are one step closer to achieving your most cherished goals!

NOTE: Spices and herbs can also be added to *your* diet menus in moderation. They do NOT add calories, but they DO enhance any type of food. Practice with some of these until your personal palate is pleased with the results. Use this as a guide toward purchasing spices for specific foods. (Of course, salt has not been listed because all but the tiniest bit of salt should be eliminated from any reducing diet.)

BAY LEAF: Aromatic leaf of a species of laurel tree grown in Mediterranean countries. Uses: *Dried,* in pickling, stews, soups; is often an ingredient in herb mixtures or the bouquet garni.

BLACK PEPPER: Peppercorns are the dried berries of the pepper vine to be ground in a mill or used in spice bags. Black pepper, the whole berry ground, has a pungent taste. Used more than any other spice, it seasons appetizers, pepper cookies, meats, poultry, fish and seafood, gravies, sauces, eggs, casseroles, soups, salads, vegetables, pickles, relishes, mixed spices and chutneys.

CAYENNE, RED and WHOLE CHILI PEPPERS: These south-of-the border favorites are all members of the capsicum family, have a piquant flavor which varies in intensity. They are used for many meat dishes, especially Mexican, sausages, dressings, gravies, sauces, casseroles, spaghettis, stews, pizzas, chicken, fish seafood, eggs, cheese, soups, salads, vegetables, pickles, relishes and chutneys.

CUMIN: Small, dried fruit (seed) resembling caraway seed in shape, from the Mediterranean Islands, Morocco and India. Uses: Largely in making chili powder for Mexican cookery, also an ingredient of curry powder.

FENNEL: Herb of the carrot family cultivated for its aromatic seeds. Uses: Seeds used with fish, in some pastries popular in Scandinavian and Italian cooking, flavors candies and liqueurs.

MACE: Fleshy growth between the nutmeg shell and outer husk, orange-red in color; flavor resembles nutmeg. From Netherlands East Indies, and Grenada, British West Indies. Uses: Blends well with fish, fish sauces, pickling, preserving, stewed cherries. *Ground,* in baked goods, pastries, pound cake; also in mashed, hashed or creamed potatoes, creamed mushrooms and various dishes.

MARJORAM: For veal, pork, beef, lamb, fowl, hash croquettes, poultry, sauces, omelets, cheese dishes, stuffings, carrots and soups.

OREGANO: Herb grown in Mexico and cultivated, known also as both *Mexican sage* and *wild sweet marjoram.* Uses: *Ground* and added to chili powder; used fresh or dry in salads, salad dressings, meat cookery.

PAPRIKA: Ground from the pods of a mild pepper with a pleasant odor, an agreeable, slightly sweet taste and bright color. Garnishes canapes and appetizers, used in and on beef, pork, veal, lamb, sausage, game, stews, goulash, fish, shellfish, poultry, egg and cheese dishes, soups, salads, and to top vegetables lacking in color.

POPPY SEED: Seed of the poppy plant, imported, largely from Holland. Uses: Topping for breads, crackers, rolls, cookies, in salads, in cheese, added to sweet fillings for pastry.

ROSEMARY: For pork, lamb, beef, veal, chicken fricassee, string beans. A sweet, minty herb, it is very strong, so go lightly. Wonderful in combination with garlic powder and parsley.

SAFFRON: Uses: Dried and powdered, it is used as coloring in rich dishes, in curry powder, in many sauces, in mustard pickles, and Oriental cookery.

SAGE: For all stuffings, sausage, roast pork, goose, dried beans, onions, tomato soup. A tiny pinch of sage and a tiny pinch of garlic powder with thyme and parsley added to canned soups is good.

SAVORY: For all bean, pea, lentil dishes, eggplant, squash. Good in stuffings of all kinds. It is more subtle than sage when used in meat balls, croquettes, meat loaf, stews.

TARRAGON: For fish, all seafood, hot or cold chicken, mushrooms, eggs, salads, sauces, spinach, celery and tomatoes.

THYME: For clam or fish chowder, all meats, fowl, stews, soup, stuffings, carrots, peas, scalloped onions, eggplant. Blends well with other herbs.

TURMERIC: Available mostly ground, this spice is the root of a plant of the ginger family and has a slightly bitter flavor. Used in recipes for cakes, cookies, curried meats, fish, shell-fish, poultry, eggs, sauces, gravies, rice, salads, dressings. Its most common uses are in curry powders, pickles, relishes, chowchows, chutneys and in condiments such as prepared mustard.

VEGETABLE SOUP

1 cup finely chopped onions
   (scallions or green
   onions are best)
2 cups green peas, or
   1 box (10 ounces)
   frozen peas
1 head lettuce, coarsely cut
1 pound spinach leaves
½ cup chopped parsley
1 teaspoon dried tarragon

or 1 tablespoon fresh
   tarragon leaves
Few leaves sorrel, if available
3 tablespoons butter or
   margarine; pinch of salt
   and pepper
2 quarts hot water
3 egg yolks
½ cup heavy cream

Sauté vegetables and herbs in butter for 2 minutes. Add 1 teaspoon salt and ⅛ teaspoon pepper. Add water and bring to boil. Cover and simmer until vegetables are just tender. Strain and keep liquid. Put vegetables through sieve or blender. Return to pot. Add ¾ of the liquid. At serving time, bring soup to boil. Beat egg yolks. Combine with remainder of liquid and the cream. Heat, gently stirring constantly. Do not boil. When mixture has thickened, stir into soup. Taste for seasoning. Serve at once.

Makes 2½ quarts, serves 6 to 8.

TOMATOES A LA HERBS

4 firm tomatoes
2 tablespoons butter
⅓ cup bread crumbs
a pinch of pepper

⅓ teaspoon salt
¼ basil leaf
½ teaspoon rosemary
   leaves (crushed)

Wash tomatoes and remove stem ends. Cut in half. Melt butter in saucepan and gently brush over cut surfaces of tomatoes. Use remaining butter to sprinkle over bread crumbs. Place crumb mixture on each tomato half. Place tomatoes under broiler (low heat—about 250 degrees). Broil for 8-10 minutes until tomatoes are heated through and crumbs are browned. Serves 4.

BAKED TOMATOES AND BASIL

1 lb. tomatoes
2 onions
1 tablespoon chopped basil

Breadcrumbs
Butter; dash of sugar, salt
   and pepper

Slice the tomatoes and onions. Put a layer of tomatoes in the bottom of a buttered pie dish, then a dessert spoon full of basil and a layer of onions. Season with salt and pepper, a sprinkling of sugar and dot lightly with butter. Repeat this until the dish is full, then top with breadcrumbs and pieces of butter. Bake in a moderate oven for 20 minutes. The aroma that greets you when this is taken from the oven is marvelous. Suggestion: Serve with roast beef or lamb.

ASPARAGUS

1 lb. asparagus	boiling water
2 oz. butter	salt, pepper

Ideally, asparagus should be cooked standing on end as the stalks take longer than the tips.

Trim the stalks, wash gently and tie in a tidy bundle. Stand in a deep jar, add a little salt, pour in boiling water two-thirds of the way up. Stand this in a pan of boiling water. Cover the pan and boil for 30 minutes. (Or fix as you usually do) . Serve with hollandaise sauce.

HOLLANDAISE SAUCE

3 egg yolks	1 tablespoon wine vinegar
2 oz. butter	salt, pepper (to season)

The secret of this sauce is that it must not ever boil; also good fresh butter must be used.

Melt the butter in a double saucepan or in a basin over hot water. Mix the egg yolks, vinegar, salt and pepper, add to the melted butter, stir briskly without stopping until the sauce is smooth and thick. Taste and add more salt and pepper if you think it needs it. Pour over asparagus.

ROSEMARY TEA

Take a sprig of rosemary and put it in a cup, pour boiling water over it, stand a saucer on the top to keep in the fumes, leave to infuse for 5 minutes. If making more than 1 cup, use several sprigs and make the tea in a teapot.

COFFEE ALA REY

Make strong, hot coffee. For each cup take one clove, a two inch piece of stick cinnamon, a small piece of orange peel and one of lemon, and a lump of sugar. Pour in one teaspoon of Martinique rum and one teaspoon of cognac. Place another lump of sugar in a tablespoon, put some of this prepared liquid over it and set it on fire, then lower it in to the rest. Add your piping hot coffee and serve.

MARINADE

The object of the marinade process is to soften and "perfume" meat prior to cooking. To make a marinade you need:

lemon juice	salt
oil	pepper
thyme	white wine or Brandy
bay leaf	(optional)
parsley	

Mix above ingredients (use your judgment on quantities dependent upon quantity of meat).

Allow meat to bathe in this "perfumed" mixture prior to cooking for at least 3 hours.

BARBECUE SAUCE SUPREME

Dice an onion and fry it in three tablespoons of butter. Add two cloves of garlic, one tablespoon of sugar, one teaspoon of salt, one teaspoon of chili powder, one teaspoon of black pepper, one tablespoon of paprika, half a tablespoon of dry mustard. Mix well. Add two cups of meat stock, one cup of vinegar, a dash of tabasco and one teaspoon of Worcestershire sauce. Simmer for an hour. Strain. Use to baste your meat.

BOUQUET GARNI
(A tiny bundle of aromatic herbs)

3 sprigs parsely (including stems)
1 sprig thyme
½ bay leaf

Ingredients are tied together in a piece of muslin which makes them easier to extract (prior to serving) after use in soups, stews, etc.

HERB SAUCE

Use a mixture of any of the following herbs:
chives, parsley, onion, watercress, fennel

olive oil
wine vinegar
salt
sugar

Quantities of ingredients will depend on the number you are serving.

Chop herbs finely. Add olive oil and wine vinegar to the consistency of a thick sauce. Add a pinch of salt and sugar to taste. Serve with buffet dishes—especially cold meats.

CANTALOUPE (CAN-ELOPE)

1 cantaloupe
2 jiggers of brandy
5 oz. Confectioner's Sugar
1 lemon (juice only)

Peel the melon, remove all tiny seeds. Cut melon into cubes. Mix brandy, lemon and sugar well. Pour mixture over melon pieces. Cover and allow melon to marinate in juice for at least three hours. Toss lightly. Can be topped with whipped cream, if desired.

BANANAS A LA CHERIE (oo la la)

2 large bananas
1 oz. sugar
⅓ pint cream
¼ pint sherry

Peel bananas and mash them through a sieve or strainer, add sugar. Stir, add cream. Beat (whipping motions) for about five minutes, or until mixture thickens. Gradually add sherry and beat. Chill for three hours.

CHERRIES A LA FLAME
(Light A Torch in His Heart)

1 can large black (pitted) cherries
1 pint French vanilla ice cream
2 tablespoons sugar
1 tablespoon cornstarch
½ cup cognac

Drain the cherries, pouring off the juice. Mix sugar and cornstarch, add just enough of the cherry juice to mixture to make a fine paste. Add this to the balance of the juice. Cook in saucepan over a a low heat. Simmer for about three minutes. Add cherries. Remove from heat. Add cognac. Ignite it with a long stemmed match. Fill sherbert or dessert dish with a scoop of French Vanilla ice cream. Allow flames to smoulder and die of their own accord.

CLARET PEARS

(How Pears become *Pairs*)

8 pears	6 cloves
4 tablespoon sugar	2/3 pint water
grated rind of 1 lemon	1/3 pint claret

Peel pears, cut in half and remove cores. Put them in a large saucepan with sugar, lemon rind, cloves, water and wine and simmer gently, covered, for 2 hours. Chill in the refrigerator and serve with whipped cream.

COQ AU VIN

1 young chicken	1 pint red wine
(cut up in 6 pieces)	bouquet garni
2 oz. butter	1 liquor glass brandy
2 oz. lean bacon	(1 jigger)
4 oz. sliced mushrooms	pepper
1 clove of garlic	

Melt the butter in a saucepan, add the diced bacon, the mushrooms, pepper. Fry all for 5 minutes till browned. Add the chopped garlic and the bouquet. Pour the brandy over and set it alight, add the wine, cover the pot and simmer for twenty minutes.

FRENCH HERBED CHICKEN

Select a 2½ - 3 lb. fryer, cut up.
Coat chicken in mixture of 1/3 cup flour,
1½ teaspoons salt and ½ teaspoon pepper
Brown chicken in skillet, in small amount of fat.

Remove chicken. In same skillet add 8 small whole onions, ½ cup coarsely chopped carrots, 1 clove of garlic, crushed. Cover and cook 5 minutes.

In tea ball or cheesecloth bag, place 4 sprigs parsley, 1 bay leaf, ¼ tsp. dried thyme leaves and 2 or 3 sprigs celery leaves. Place in large casserole. Add chicken, cooked vegetables, one 3 oz. can sliced mushrooms in layers.

Add 2 cups red Burgundy to same skillet; heat, scrape up browned pieces from bottom and pour over casserole. Cover. Bake in 350° oven 2 hours.

CINNAMON BREAD

Take slices of bread, remove the crusts, and cut into strips. Toast one side to a light brown. Cream four tablespoons of butter and spread on the hot, untoasted side. Mix four tablespoons of powdered sugar with three of cinnamon and sprinkle over the buttered side. Put back in the oven until sugar is melted. Serve in a covered dish at once.

HERB OMELET

Serves 4
  6 eggs
  3 teaspoons—chopped parsley
  4 sprigs—fresh parsley
  3 teaspoons—fresh chopped chives
  2 tablespoons (smoothed off) butter
  black pepper
  salt
  1 teaspoon water

Mix eggs in bowl preferably with a fork (but do *not* beat). Add parsley, chives, seasonings and water to eggs. Melt butter in frying pan. Pour in egg mixture as soon as butter gets hot. When eggs begin to set raise sides of omelet with a fork to enable uncooked portion to slide under. While mixture is still a bit runny on top, fold it over and serve immediately. The whole cooking process should take only a few minutes.

Part VI

Life Is a Gift—Take It!

*It is part of the cure
to wish to be cured.*

—SENECA

The Beauty Pavilion

Within recent months, my Beauty Pavilion has made quite a name for itself. One reporter, on examining the building, opined that the structure could not help but become the beauty center of the world! I was indeed both pleased and flattered, pleased because this reporter had recognized a dream of mine turned into something tangible; flattered because anyone else understanding my dream was fulfilling the first necessary step.

For years, I have carried the blueprints for a complete beauty hospital around in my head. For a long time I had envisioned a special goal: to bring together, under one roof, a completely equipped beauty hospital featuring all the latest in plastic and cosmetic surgery techniques for the beautification of all who seek same.

Today, that vision is a reality! The Beauty Pavilion is a rotunda-shaped edifice containing ten thousand square feet of space dedicated to beauty. Within the Pavilion we have housed a TOTAL SCIENTIFIC approach to beauty. It is the only clinical facility in the country dedicated *exclusively* to beauty.

The stress on beauty begins the moment a patient

191

enters the front door of The Pavilion, but it will NOT end when she goes home. In addition to any surgery or other treatment performed, each patient can be given a private consultation with beauty experts in other fields. She will take away with her not only a NEW LOOK but a *lasting approach* to the maintenance of beauty.

Among the other cosmetic surgery techniques being employed at The Beauty Pavilion, there is a new technique, available for the first time. I call this technique MINI-MAX—it is actually a new fast way for a person to avail herself of the beauty treatments. Heretofore, a patient required a *series* of procedures to complete the improvement desired. Now, I have come up with streamlined versions of facial procedures which can be completed in minutes, require no hospitalization, patients being up and around immediately.

To give you an example, because of the techniques perfected and the employment of the newest facilities, a patient can arrive at The Beauty Pavilion on Friday, have her nose bobbed, bags under the eyes eliminated, wrinkles removed from her face, the size and firmness of her breasts taken care of, and she can be on her way home BEFORE the weekend is over!

Because of the methods used in The Beauty Pavilion, a woman can have a complete "Beauty Weekend" no matter where she resides. One can board a plane in New York, arrive in Los Angeles, enter The Beauty Pavilion, go through a complete consultation, and actually have everything required performed, and re-board her homeward bound plane within forty-eight hours!

So, you have been introduced to my Beauty Pavilion . . . and now, for the balance of this Chapter, I will answer the questions put to me most frequently when patients write to me at the Pavilion.

The morning mail looks something like this:

Robert Alan Franklyn, M.D.
The Beauty Pavilion
8760 Sunset Boulevard
Los Angeles, California 90069.
Dear Dr. Franklyn:

I am only thirty years of age yet I have bags under my eyes, making me look like "The Morning After." What can be done about this?

Simple eyelifts take but a few minutes to perform and heal without a trace in two days time. The excess bagginess is removed through a tiny incision just at the edge of the lid, with the patient resuming activity the same morning.

At thirty-four years of age I seem to have lost the bloom of youth and my face looks droopy. Am I too young for a face lift?

You can use a mini-lift instead of the more effective regular face lifts which are required when the neck begins to droop also. The mini-lift is a fifteen minute procedure, hidden within the temple area of the scalp, so as not to be noticeable. This gently lifts and supports the cheeks of the thirties giving a regained sparkle.

Is the soft gel implant method for breast enlargement simpler than breast injections?

Breast enlargement by means of a smooth, soft, contoured implant behind the breast, is the best method. This may take as little as ten minutes to perform in actual operating time, achieving an instant and permanent, beautiful new full shape. Injections are uneven, require many treatments and do not last.

At what ages do peoples' faces begin to break down?

First the eyes become baggy and then the cheeks droop

a bit, with groove lines appearing between the nose and the corners of the mouth. The can be corrected in the thirties by eye lifts and miniature face lifts. Later the jaw line becomes jowly and the neck skin loosens and sags. This then requires a routine face lift, done mainly behind the ears, into the hairline behind the neck. All of these beauty procedures are done in a matter of minutes with local novocaine, so that the patient is up and about the same morning and back to activity. Modern procedures are streamlined compared to the old days of general anesthetics and weeks in a hospital!

Do you advise facial massages? Must they be professionally given, or are there ways to do it at home?

Yes, I do advise the principle of facial massage, and this, too, can be done at home. Without in the least selling short either the physical benefits or psychological joys of relaxing under the skilled fingers of a professional masseuse, you can, and should, be able to do this for yourself.

You see, your face has more than fifty muscles. The fibers are interwoven and work together as teams when you laugh, or cry, or smile, or frown. These muscles are attached to the inner layer of your skin and need regular perking up. Massage helps to bring color and pink freshness to the face, helps strengthen sagging facial muscles, and stirs up blood circulation.

Before massage, the face should always be cleaned, either by simple washing, or through a steaming process. For the latter, (if you do not own a home-style Sauna facial steamer) cover your head and shoulders with a large towel and drape the towel over a bowl of freshly boiled water into which you have added the juice of a fresh lemon. The simplest form of facial massage is done with a thin film of nourishing cream. First cleanse skin thoroughly. Apply and knead cream gently into the face. Work from your chin to your jawline, and up from the bottom of your cheeks to the top. Apply across your upper lip and massage along the nose. Working from the center of your forehead toward your temples, massage gently. Pat expression lines from mouth to nose and upward on the forehead from eyebrows to the hair line. Be careful—do not stretch the skin with the patting movements. Remove any remaining cream with a tonic lotion and follow with an astringent.

My skin is oily and it never seems to be free of blackheads. Can you give me a few clues on the treatment and care of blackheads?

Oily skin has many blessings, but it also carries with it a few drawbacks, or at least some problem areas which require special attention and care.

Both blackheads *and* whiteheads are problems associated with oily skin. Blackheads are concentrations of dirt that mix with the oil to build unsightly masses in the pores. Whiteheads are concentrations of the oil itself.

The problem is often the result of poor circulation. Absolute cleanliness and frequent facial scrubbing helps, but be careful not to damage skin tissue. The friction from moistened grainy cereal is also helpful in dislodging blackheads. Scrubbing will not always remove whiteheads, however. If they are too deeply entrenched in your skin, you may need medical assistance.

Try a coarse washcloth or complexion brush, use a rotary motion in cleansing your face. Brush or scrub most vigorously in the places where the oil tends to gather—your hairline, nose creases and chin. After rinsing with clear water, pat your face dry and work in an astringent.

Is there a do-it-yourself formula for your Cosmo-Face Pack which I can follow in my own home?

Yes, here is a home-made version of the Cosmo-Face Pack treatment that uses the same oils I use on bandages which cover the sutures of plastic surgery. These oils have a high degree of natural antibiotic quality. A skin treated with these oils resists any harmful effects from the sun, while retaining the good effects. A face treated with the Cosmo-Pack retains make-up without fading or "running." That is one reason why the treatment is so popular in Hollywood.

To prepare your own Cosmo-Face Pack take bay, eucalyptus, aloe, or any other such leaves you especially like. Bay leaves, of course, are commonly found right in your own kitchen, as are marjoram, oregano, and other spices from the vast array of aromatics. Add four ounces of prepared tea (not leaves.) Fill up an electric blender. Liquify to a consistency thick enough to adhere to the skin. Store in a dark place for several days. After applying, lie down and relax for fifteen minutes. Remove with tepid water.

A friend of mine told me she was advised to make a facial using Sea Salts. Is this preparation really good for the skin?

Definitely—if used properly. You can buy Sea Salt at health-food stores, and in some drug stores, and give yourself a facial right at home. In fact it is very easy. Make a pack of your Sea Salts by mixing salts with warm water until it is the consistency of moist sand. Before applying, sauna steam your face a bit, or apply hot towels for a few minutes. You can leave the pack on for about fifteen minutes. However, if you want to give yourself the touch of a professional treatment, lie down and apply hot towels to your face while the pack is on.

The Sea Salt pack has been called a "remodeling massage" because it "wipes off weariness and wrinkles." It will not only give your skin a lovely freshness, but the salt has a tightening effect and is truly a "remodeling massage." So relax and let it work for you.

Lately I have had trouble with my skin. Can you tell me what dermabrasion is, and is it usually effective?

Whatever your skin troubles, there are modern techniques which are excellent means of defense against the aging appearance of the skin. Aesthetic surgery can do wonders in rejuvenation by tightening the lax skin of the face and thus restoring a youthful smoothness. Then, there is another method which requires no surgery. This is dermabrasion.

Dermabrasion, as practiced by the specialists, consists of applications of a spinning diamond wheel which removes a layer of the epidermis. Since the skin conditions and qualities differ from person to person, each subject must be treated individually. The specialists of this method of rejuvenating the skin have made profound studies of the many skin types and they vary their treatments accordingly.

The surface is skimmed off. Under this tired surface lies new, smooth, unblemished skin that will soon replace the old skin. But once the new skin is exposed, it must be cared for because it is very delicate.

However, for the ravages of age, the droop and excess skin, the simplest process is the *temple face lift* which takes but twenty minutes to do and is hidden within the temple areas of the scalp. This is often done in conjunction with an injection or two of the Cleopatra's Needle to plump out the sunken lines and hollows of the face which often precede the droopy face.

The process of aging usually becomes visible when a woman reaches twenty-six or twenty-seven, and then bags begin to appear under the eyes. As a woman gets older she acquires puffy areas and loose skin on her face. If these are attended to early enough, one only requires a minor eye lift in which the excess skin and puffs are removed. The operation—which takes only fifteen to twenty minutes—is very satisfying in terms of results achieved. In this operation, the excess baggy skin is removed. Within three days the area is almost devoid of all signs of any surgery and is the fastest healing of all operations.

As a woman ages, her cheeks tend to droop around the eye area. At twenty-nine or thirty deep lines or grooves usually appear between the nose and the mouth. In this instance, the Cleopatra's Needle technique works on eliminating these facial grooves. Also, a minor temple lift is sufficient here, too. However, if a woman allows herself to reach her late forties, or fifties, or even her sixties without taking advantage of a minor eye lift or a temple lift, then a major face lift may be in order.

If a major face lift is required, this, too, is a relatively uncomplicated procedure from the patient's point of view. A major face lift requires about forty-five minutes of surgery and is done around and behind the ears. In this operation the excess skin from the neck and face is smoothed upward and removed, requiring only a number of tiny stitches which are removed within seven to ten days.

All of the operations and facial improvements I have mentioned are done with a local anesthetic and with the patient in a sitting up position. No hospitalization is required. A patient comes in during the morning and can leave that *same* morning under her own power.

I've always been embarrassed by the shape of my breasts. I understand this a common problem and one for which there are various forms of "help" available. Who do you advise?

First of all, let me assure you that yours is indeed a common problem. In fact, eighty out of one hundred women, regardless of age, suffer mental and emotional agonies over what they consider imperfect breasts. This "torment" is no longer necessary. Even the most unendowed woman can acquire bosom beauty through various methods of remedying shape and size. Without getting too technical, let me just say that the shape of the breasts involves such elements as glands, tissue, skin and muscles. The muscles are of two types: the underlying ones are the large and small pectorals; over these are the second type, the superficial surface muscles. The pectorals are *voluntary* muscles. The superficial ones are *involuntary* and will react only to stimuli such as temperature change or electric currents. Both sets of muscles must be considered since both contribute to the breasts' firmness. To aid muscles, you must exercise.

Here are some exercises I recommend:

A. Lying face down, support your body on your hands and toes. Raise your body up, then lower it. Do these pushups as long as you can and, at all times, keep the body rigid.

If you have trouble mastering this fairly difficult movement, start by holding onto the arm of a chair and, in a leaning position, push your stiffened body to and from the chair.

B. Stand erect. Hold your hands together, palm-to-palm. Now—as if you were trying to flatten something between your hands—use the force of your arms to press your hands together. Do this from twenty to fifty times.

C. Sit before a table. Form your hands into fists. Place your fists on the table so that your breasts and your fists are aligned. Now, press with all your force against your fists—hold it a few seconds and then relax. Repeat at least fifty times.

D. Roll up a bath towel, and then twist it as if you were trying to wring water from it. Put all your force into the movement, and repeat from twenty to forty times in a row. Breathe deeply between each movement.

These exercises will not correct breast defects, but they can contribute to form and firmness of your breasts.

Breast beauty, granted by nature, or created or improved by surgery, can be helped by exercise. However, all the exercise in the world will not cure the flat or droopy breast for which simple surgery is still the instant answer.

Although I am not really overweight, I am self-conscious about the thickness of my neck. I feel I look top-heavy. Have you any advice for me?

Well, according to theory, the distance around your neck should be equal to the circumference of your knee, half of the circumference of your waist, and twice the circumference of your wrist. If your neck measurements do not meet this test, do not be disheartened. You can make improvements. The neck should be graceful and shapely, a lovely pivot for the head. However too often it is anything but a thing of beauty and mainly because of neglect.

To achieve a graceful appearance you should exercise your neck. Not only will this improve your physical appearance but it will also help to improve your circulation, fortify your muscles and render the tissues more supple. Rotating the head or swiveling it from side-to-side, leaning the head forward as far as possible are all excellent limbering exercises, but they should be practiced with maximum effort. Also, you should massage your neck just as conscientiously as you do your face, with nourishing products and hydrating lotions. There are also special products for double chins and for cleansing the throat tissues. When you massage the chin, always stroke downward. Also, using the tips of the fingers, massage with a circular motion; using the left hand for the right side and the right hand for the left side. Tapping the neck with cotton saturated in tonic lotion and spraying it with cold water is also a helpful practice.

Become consciously aware of your bearing. Carry your head up, your shoulders straight; don't allow your head to sag when writing or reading, and don't destroy the contours of your face by leaning your chin heavily on your hand. I believe these few simple exercises, plus frequent beauty treatments, will help you solve your problem.

Once the neck has become loose and crepy, the face lined and jowly, do not expect much from exercises or gadgets. A morning spent at the plastic surgery clinic is needed to shed the excess droopy skin.

Is there a way to tighten facial skin once it starts to sag?

Unfortunately there is no miraculous means of making skin taut once it becomes flaccid, although a great deal of research has been poured into the problem. But the research *has led* to the discovery of skin-tightening aids of diverse organs: vegetal (citrus juices, witch hazel, tannin) and animal (nearly all serums). These aids are found in creams and lotions that are helpful for stimulating the tonicity of the skin.

A natural astringent, which is not as efficacious as the prepared products, is ice, or cold water. It affects muscle fibre, causing it to contract, bringing about a temporary tightening of tissue. Constant repetitive application is necessary to keep the surface taut.

Medical science also has contributed aids for eliminating sagging skin, such as peeling, dermabrasion and needle therapy. To answer briefly, the point is that skin need not sag and drag away beauty provided you have taken care of yourself religiously starting at an early age.

As sad as sagging skin seems, it is a relatively mild telegraphic warning compared to such cries for help as acne, dandruff herpes and other blemishes. These stand on the skin's surface like glaciers: as ugly as they look on the surface, you can be sure there is a lot more trouble down below, whereas with simple sag and aging, swift face lifting is the answer.

I'm a very active person—or at least I try to be. Lately my feet are letting me down—and getting me down. What can I do to help myself? I'm a salesperson required to stand for many hours each day.

There could be many reasons for excessive fatigue and aching feet. For example, one of the most common abuses of the feet is wearing shoes selected for *style* rather than comfort, causing ingrown toenails, corns, bunions, and even bone deformation. In fact, these conditions can be aggravated to a point where the only corrective measure is an operation.

While high heels may be worn for elegant occasions, shoes made for walking or working in should be half-heels, or very low ones. Sandals and ballet slippers should get part-time wear since they offer little support for the foot.

Massage your feet with special creams and lotions. Keep your toenails trimmed properly and visit a pedicurist periodically. Your feet will feel better, and serve you better. Also you might try these exercises:

A. Stand with your feet about five inches apart. Slowly lift your heels until you are balancing on the balls of your feet and on your toes. Descend extremely slowly.

B. Walk in your bare feet around a room, walking on the edges of your feet, first on the outside edge and then inside. Stop occasionally to pick up a pencil from the floor with your toes.

C. Sit on a chair. Extend your feet before you. Point the toes forward as far as possible, then point them up and back toward you as far as possible. Repeat ten times.

My hands always seem so much drier than the skin on the rest of my body. Is there a reason for this? Can you advise any special hand care?

The skin of your hands *is* apt to be dryer than that of your face and the rest of your body because the skin on your hands has fewer oil cells. Therefore hands *do* need special care. They need a soap rich in lanolin, they need protective covering, and they need special care routines to replace lost moisture.

The nails need calcium, Vitamin B and proteins for health. If these elements are missing in the body, your health suffers. Therefore, the nails serve as a sign of health deficiencies. Proper diet and vitamin-intake, plus care, can enhance the shiny transparency and the smooth surface of the nails.

There are many household and professional tasks

that can impair the beauty of hands, especially if the hands come in contact with irritating products, such as some detergents which can cause excessive dryness.

In dishwashing, there is another enemy along with detergent—hot water. Therefore, for good hand care: first, don't use very hot water; second, try wearing rubber gloves when you do dishes. Third, there are numerous hand care products on the market for your use. In fact, it is a good idea to keep a jar of hand cream, or a dispenser of hand lotion at various locations in your home wherever you might wash your hands, especially near your kitchen sink. If you are a professional or business person, take some hand lotion to work with you. Carry a tube of hand cream in your pocketbook. This special attention definitely will pay off.

Can a flabby abdomen really be corrected by plastic surgery?

Yes, only I like to label this procedure, along with other surgical improvements of face and body, BEAUTY SURGERY. Operations for remodeling the abdomen are often performed to remove unsightly abdominal bulges which are the result of fat tissue or flabby skin. Even rolls of fat around the midriff can be removed by surgery. This is done by drawing the tissues and skin of the waist region up, and making them taut.

Is there any at-home treatment for thinning hair?

In giving yourself a hot oil treatment, the scalp must first be massaged from 7 to 10 minutes, to bring up the circulation. A hair oil is then applied to the scalp warm, with a cotton pledget. Separating the hair, strand by strand, will help in getting the oil to the scalp. Wring a turkish towel in very hot water and wrap around head. Use several hot towels. This forces the oil into the scalp and the hair roots. Do not shampoo for approximately thirty minutes. Dry hair by hand and before completely dry, apply ointment or pomade to scalp. This will serve to heal the scalp if inclined to sensitiveness from the treatment.

My hands look awful although I do take care of them. I have a problem with breakage—my nails split so easily. What can you advise?

A hot oil treatment is excellent for nails that are brittle or that split and break easily. Another important step is to remove nail polish and to keep it off for several days during the first series of treatments. Select one night a week when it is possible for you to be without nail polish. Remove your polish and give yourself an oil treatment. To do that, heat a portion of vegetable oil and soak your fingertips for twenty minutes Wipe the fingers dry with absorbent cotton—*be sure to leave a coating of oil on your nails.* During the first series of treatments, dab a bit of oil on your nails as often as possible during the day.

After your nail condition has improved, an occasional oil treatment should do. You might also apply white iodine once a week to your polish-free nails to make them stronger.

Be sure that all your manicure products have an oily base. Nail polish remover can make your nails brittle unless it is of the oily variety.

Diet plays an important part in fingernail strength. Make sure you acquire plenty of protein through lean meat, eggs, fish and milk. The "B for Beauty" vitamin-intake is also important. Ask your own physician about the advisability of increasing your calcium intake via calcium tablets, at least until your nails grow harder.

Is there any routine or ritual for maintaining a healthy scalp?

Yes. Daily brushing and massage are the first ingredients in any prescription for a healthy scalp.

In order for your scalp to be healthy, those oil glands must be well-regulated and must have freely-circulating blood.

If your scalp tends to be dry, you should massage vigorously for greater stimulation of the tiny oil glands. If it tends to oilness, massage gently. In either case, massage with your fingertips, or with a gentle vibrator.

A. Hand-massage should be performed with all ten fingers. Use the cushions at your fingertips to massage in tiny circles, from the nape of your neck to the top of your head. Pay special attention to the hairlines.

B. Next, starting on the area just above your ears, massage in small circles to the top of your head.

C. Finally, knead the top of your scalp.

If you do these three steps every day your scalp will stay healthy and you will feel vigorous, alive and free from tension.

NOTE: If your scalp is unusually dry, you might try the above exercises employing a dab of hair tonic to each of the steps.

Could you please explain the process and purpose of face peeling?

Peeling is the application of chemical agents to the outer layers of skin, thereby removing disfigurements. It is a branch of therapy also known as *cosmetic chemo-surgery.*

As practiced by specialists, peeling consists of applying a preparation which removes a layer of the outer skin, the epidermis. This causes the skin to loosen, permitting the surface to be peeled right off and reveal smooth, unblemished skin that is as fine as a baby's.

The use of peeling, however, must be decided on an individual basis. Since the skin condition and qualities differ from one person to another, each peeling subject must be treated individually. Treatments even vary for the various parts of the face.

In summary, peeling isn't a quick miracle. There are specific conditions to be met for peeling to be successful. A woman of advanced years, for example, shouldn't hope for an immediate return of her youthful face with just the first peeling. The specialists, to do a successful job, will make a careful study of the changes on each section of the face, to determine whether to use chemical or surgical methods.

There have been more stunning results where facial wrinkles, crow's-feet, and crepy necks have been "peeled" away by surgical means such as face lifting rather than by chemical peeling.

I have seen many "beauty products" advertised which stress the use of various fruits and vegetables in their ingredients. Is there any validity to preparations of this type or is this just another sales gimmick?

While of course, I am unable to endorse or even suggest commercial beauty products by name, in general I can tell you that there is a very definite historical basis for the use of fruits and such in beauty preparations. You see, man's use of the elements around him—plants, herbs, fruits—goes back beyond material medica and pharmacology.

We find pictorial records of Assyrian and Egyptian slaves using freshly-gathered fruits to prepare beauty masks for their mistresses.

In ancient Rome the juice of the grape, the apple and other fruits were used for skin culture.

Then, as organic chemistry grew, man began to de-emphasize the natural and concentrate on the synthetic.

But today modern research has run the full circle and is back to accentuating the natural forces inherent in the fruits of the earth, the life forces of growing things. Grape is used today in anti-wrinkle creams and in beauty masks. Strawberry is included in cleansing cream, skin tonics, astringents and skin lotions. Orange is found in emollients or soothing lotions and in cleansing creams. Lemon is used in skin whiteners, skin fresheners and skin tonics. Thus you see, that while I am unable to discuss specific commercial beauty preparations, I can at least confirm that the proper use of nature's products can indeed be helpful. You will find do-it-yourself formulas for such products throughout this book.

I have heard that sun-tanning on the beach can be advantageous. Is this so?

You have heard correctly. But first, a word of warning. Moderation is the key. While it may seem foolish to admonish the adult not to over-do sun-tanning, at the beach, or elsewhere, the *proper* use of sun, sea and sand can indeed be therapeutic. Therefore, assuming you realize the danger of repeated prolonged over-exposure to the sun's rays, I will now get to your specific question.

Sunning at the beach may provide a healthy plus besides sun—the sand. Sand has a proven therapeutic quality, and it should be taken advantage of. Try "burying" yourself with it. You will find your body will perspire copiously without you being aware of it. The burying process is something like taking a Turkish bath without the discomfort of the hot steam.

Take a sand bath from ten minutes to half an hour. As the perspiration is absorbed by the dry sand, your glands will produce more—and all the time your body is "washing out" its toxic substances.

As your body perspires, your capillary vessels dilate, sending blood circulating and coursing through your body, refreshing it, stimulating it. While the experience is similar to a Turkish bath, in the sand bath you are also gaining health benefits while just lying and relaxing.

Sand serves as a sedative, aside from its role as a stimulant. It tends to penetrate the aches and pains, thus soothing your nerves.

So the combination of sun and sand when employed in moderation is indeed very advantageous.

To achieve lasting beauty, you must want it, work for it, live it every day of your life. The suggestions throughout this book can quickly become like second nature to you—try them and become a new you!

Breastplasty

Judging from the great number of questions I am asked and the letters which I receive, the appearance of the breasts obviously is a major preoccupation. It would seem that many times the size of breasts and their firmness are the principal factors for making a woman happy or unhappy. In a great number of cases, the problems are exaggerated, especially in view of the fact that modern brassieres can give an ideal appearance. Even so, one should not overlook or neglect any possibilities of beautifying the breasts and correcting any existing faults. For this, there are any number of perfected treatments which are beneficial if one does not demand the impossible.

Because of the structure of the breasts (glands encased in fat tissue and sustained by elastic fibers and skin), they are very fragile. Their development and firmness is governed by hormone secretions which can be modified because of various conditions. The variation in hormone secretion in turn causes variations in the condition of the breasts.

When the enveloping tissue of the breasts lose their tensile properties the breasts sag. This condition, known as ptosis, may be due to a number of reasons: aging, loss of weight, illness (infections, nerves, digestive troubles), nursing a child, glandular upsets, etc. Once the cause has been isolated and treated, there are then many methods for re-establishing the tonicity of the breasts. For instance, the application of astringents and cold water treatments are an aid to making the dermal structure more firm. Regaining lost pounds, in cases of underweight, will help to fill out the breasts.

The muscles of the breasts are of two sorts: the underlying ones are the large and small pectorals; over these are the superficial surface muscles. The pectorals are voluntary muscles, while the superficial ones are involuntary and will only react to stimuli such as temperature change or electric currents. For the retention of the breasts' firmness the traction of the superficial muscles is more important than that of the pectoral muscles. If you study yourself in a mirror you will see that, by contracting your pectoral muscles, the effects on the breasts are negligible compared to bathing the breasts with cold water. But, since both sets of muscles contribute to the firmness of the breasts, they must both be given full consideration and attention. Exercises which require minimum arm movement are, in my opinion, best for the breasts because these are less apt to be brusquely straining to the mammary glands. Following are a few excellent excercises for the breasts:

1. Lying face down, support the body on the hands and the toes and lower and raise the body. Do this as long as possible and, at all times, keep the body rigid. If this is difficult for you to do, begin first by holding onto the arms of a chair and, in a leaning position, push your stiffened body to and from the chair.

2. Learn to control to perfection whatever movements of physical culture you undertake. You can best do this by first

practicing in front of a mirror. Concentrate on doing the movements gracefully, rapidly and effectively. It is your concentration and control which will direct the effects of the exercises to whichever part of the body you wish to modify.

3. Persistence. Only through consistent effort can you achieve a visible modifying of a body condition. It is best to limit your exercise sessions to ten to fifteen minute periods. It is wiser and better to realize your goal little by little rather than to exhaust your efforts in a few bursts of enthusiasm. Only by keeping at it can you establish a habit that will produce your desired results.

If you are one of those women who feel exercise and diet cannot improve your breasts to the extent you desire, we then come to another possible solution which can only be considered on a very personal and individual basis.

There are women with small breasts which sag, either from age, or more often than not, as a result of maternity. Both age and maternity will cause a flaccidity of the breast muscles and glands. In both cases a treatment is devised which will increase the volume of the breasts. And, in the second case, corrective measures will be taken in order to make the breasts firmer and stop their sagging. Increase of the gland volume is done by plastic surgery.

To elaborate, despite all the operations my colleagues and I have performed to bring bosoms to full beauty, the ratio still seems to remain that seven out of ten women suffer from underdeveloped breasts, in the view of our present bosom culture.

In the general sense, it seems misplaced to use the word "suffer," because there is nothing physically painful about it. But suffer they do, and acutely. It is axiomatic, at this date, to say that I have seen everything from broken marriages to attempted suicides because of the lack of what is considered today the prime female endowment.

A doctor, especially one who deals with aesthetics, likes

to see a symmetrical balance of the body—one part in harmony with the other. But today's breast cult is so pronounced that a female's figure is judged by—well, if I may
borrow that old cigarette commercial, it's certainly true
that it's what's up front that counts.

Never mind the legs, or any other part: the big question
is, is she shapely? And it means just one thing. There is a
still young actress, just past her thirtieth birthday, who it
seems to me has built her reputation as a great beauty
mostly on the size of her breasts. Her face could be considered by some to be lovely, and her coloring is something
special. But her legs are very so-so, and she hasn't the
long-boned build considered as the basis for glamor. However, she has had, since early development, a bosom that
you can't miss, and I do believe that, with a slight variance
there, she would not have acquired that reputation for
beauty that has sent men into a swoon at the mention of
her name.

Now, should there come a time when that much-vaunted
part of this famous anatomy showed a tendency to droop,
there is an operation that corrects that, too, and many
famous names have been so aided. When you see on the
screen a renowned body that was lushly endowed suddenly
take on a trim bosom, can there be any other answer?

But the more pressing problem, by far, is not the subtraction but the addition that is earnestly sought. When an
article published more than twelve years ago still brings in
mail from women in this country and other parts of the
world, I know that they are eager for facts about "the
breast operation".

That particular article showed for the first time in pic-
tures an operation performed by me to remold flat-chested
females. I'll try to answer the main points of how it's done.

It isn't only a matter of size, but of shape. The operation is the answer for women whose problem is small

breasts, from failure of development or loss of size following childbearing. My interest in breastplasty goes back
some few years, when I began to search for a substance
that would be ideal for augmenting the tissues without
disadvantages. The material I sought had to be workable.
I wanted to achieve a method of aesthetically created
breasts which would have permanency.

The latest development is a transparent synthetic jell
which looks and feels as soft as Jello. This substance,
inserted behind the breasts, will not disappear. It is easy to
do—and permanent.

In this regard, one frequently asked question is: Can a
woman who has had the breast operation nurse her
babies? This answer is simple:

"Of course." The change is *not* functional, merely aesthetic. The implant does not affect the breast tissue itself
in any way. It goes behind the glandular tissue in a small
pocket that seems almost made for it. Neither does the
operation cut into the delicate structure of the breast.
What the foam or jell does is to push the breast upward,
giving it its permanent, full curve.

What is the technique of the breastplasty operation?

Actually, it is quite simple. I make an incision with a
special, tiny knife, in the lower fold of the breasts. The
transparent synthetic jell is folded into a little ball and
inserted through the incision behind the glandular tissue.
Once inside, it curls open like a flower from the bud,
behind the breast. A few nylon stitches close the incision
line and the bandage is placed over that.

The operation is a short one—usually only ten minutes—but many things must be taken into consideration
to give a woman the result that should be truly her own.
The elasticity of skin is not uniform; body tissue varies
with the individual; skin tones and other factors must
enter into a really satisfying result. The implant must be

shaped and inserted in such a way as to provide not only the increase in measurement but also natural-looking contours that belong to the individual.

Of course, it's often the woman with a thirty-two inch bust who wants to go to a forty-two. I try to get her to accept Dr. Franklyn's "Breast Quotient" instead, to determine what size she should be. This is actually a mathematical equation worked out according to frame and height. The rest is up to the beauty surgeon, who must also be a good sculptor as well.

Where is it done?

If I do it, it is done in my Beauty Pavilion. You see, I do not believe that breastplasty requires hospitalization. It shouldn't take more than fifteen minutes, in the hands of an experienced surgeon, and the patient can leave the same day.

One advantage is in having an operating room designed especially for this surgery as I do at my Beauty Pavilion. I have a special air conditioning under negative ionization, a method by which a negative electrical charge is thrown through the air, filtering out germ and dust particles. Too, we work under powerful ultraviolet light, which sterilizes the air in the operating room as well as the skin of the patient while we are operating, this being a development of Duke University Medical School and Hospital. Recent additions are the new ozone generators, cleansing the air and sterilizing through the well-known action of ozone.

My advice to patients is to take only a few days off from work following surgery. The advantages of getting right up I have found to be enormous. It is best to keep the bandages on for a week or more. This is an elastic type which takes the place of a brassiere. At the end of this period the bandages are removed, and a new brassiere can be worn—of a larger size, naturally! Notice, I said, "can" be. I have found that many of my patients not only throw away the falsies but do not go on a buying spree for new, larger supporting bras. After all, now their support is built right in. Of course, a bra can be worn as pretty lingerie, but that's all it may be needed for!

The breastplasty operation is by no means used only because a woman wants to increase her bust measurement. It has been used to fill out breasts depleted by operations for a benign tumor, or build up similar deficiencies in what would otherwise be a hopeless situation.

Incidentally, I find it strange that so many women approach the idea of the operation with ambivalence. As much as they want results, they are bothered by the thought, "Will I be embarrassed by suddenly appearing with this new endowment?"

The fact is, because of the falsie and other secret aids that most women still employ today, the patient will probably not look too different in ordinary street clothes—but she will look better. Unless, of course, she wants to go from size thirty-two to forty-two! But in décolletage—bathing suits to evening gowns—that's where she'll happily show the difference.

Anyway, I have repeatedly had husbands bring their wives to me to become endowed. If he's not embarrassed, why should she be?

One thing is certain. There is nothing, from mechanical developers, to hormones, to exercise, that will appreciably alter the size of the breast. Exercise can improve it, by strengthening the under structure, but not enlarge it.

This is simple to understand, because the breast is not a muscle. It is composed of tissue and fat. If the fat is not there, fortunately we have found a workable replacement, the results of which I have seen alter women and their lives!

The techniques I have discussed are great "weapons" to use in your desire to "Play the Beauty Game."

I have heard a reference made to the "Cleopatra's Needle" technique. Could you explain what it does for you?

Yes. One of the most spectacular new developments in the world of beauty surgery is NOT surgery at all. No incision is made. No skin is clipped away. No stitches are taken. No bandages are used. There is no operating room or hospitalization required.

This dramatic form of "plastic surgery" is a method of simple injection of a pure solution of replacement medical silicone fluids into the subcutaneous layers of the skin where signs of aging (loss of the subcutaneous "baby fat" layer) occurs. It is a method of treating the signs of aging without a scalpel.

Injections have been used to treat the facial grooves of early advancing age, frown lines, sunken lines under the eyes, plus correcting bony hands, bony ribs and shoulders and a number of problems for which plastic surgery itself had no answers in the past. And, unlike plastic surgery, instead of cutting into the defect, injections work on the principle of repadding the tissue themselves. In our era of scientific quests for obliterating signs of advancing years, this could well be called the "secret weapon" of old age.

By means of injecting at the sight of the problem, two results are achieved: the skin is immediately plumped out, and the continous process of loss of fat cushion under the skin is retarded. Facial contours become more firm, youthful and pleasing.

Like all scientific achievements, injections are no overnight development. In fact, the discovery, like so many others, is the result of a search for an answer to catastrophe, and many international researchers have worked on the problem.

After I described this technique in a medical journal a few years ago, many other scientists did pioneer work in this field, among whom are Ludwig Lenz, of Cairo, Fumio Umezawa of Tokyo's Iui-Jin Hospital, and other Japanese investigators such as Tochiro Akiyama of Osaka Medical College, and Dr. Kamio of Tokyo, who has tested clinically silicone material in thousands of cases.

Recently medical publications have reported enthusiastic results on the injectable silicones for facial wrinkles following extensive research by different groups.

It is reported by the Dow-Corning Center for Aid to Medical Research that when the medical-grade 100 per cent pure silicones are used the body is said to be unaware that they are present. As silicone, medical fluid can even be injected into the eyeball itself to repair detached retinas safely; this is an indication of its value even in very sensitive areas.

After many years of personal work and experience with thousands of injections, following my initial report in the famous European surgical journal *Zentralblatt fur Chirurgie*, I am convinced of its value in facial and bony-hand cases. In the report referred to, material was contained which in part stimulated the European, Egyptian, and Japanese plastic surgeons previously mentioned. Pure medical-grade silicones are best in variable series of injections for extended effect, with possible occasional booster injections as time passes on.

So, "Cleopatra's Needle" is a startling development, a new phase in the entire history of plastic and cosmetic surgery. For years, plastic surgeons have been searching for something that would replace the diminished subcutaneous fatty tissue of the skin.

Surgical face lifting is a subtraction, in which excess skin is removed and the remaining skin pulled tighter. But there is more of a biophysical problem than the refitting of this "over-size" skin.

The real answer, of course, would be to replace the elasticity of the skin by renewing the worn-out tissue, achieving the original youthful firmness as part of the biological process itself, but also by restoring the lost "baby fat" layers under the skin. As we grow older and lose such padding, along comes the sagging skin and aging signs.

In advanced cases, where surgery is necessary to remove excess skin, the second step is to plump out the skin to youthful contours.

For patients of thirty to forty who are still ahead of the need for major plastic surgery, it was a revolutionary answer. They could be made to look years younger without resorting to major surgery or by combining a minor temple lift with the silicone injections.

Thus the "Cleopatra's Needle" technique (which I named in honor of work done by Dr. Lenz in Cairo, Egypt) is an advance in simplifying procedures which now can be performed in the doctor's office without hospitalization.

It is now commonplace to correct receding chins, fill out bony shoulders, and plump out wrinkled hands. Injections, in selected cases, accomplish what even plastic surgery itself has been unable to do. For instance, hand rejuvenation; it is now possible, with a few small injections, to plump out bony, tired and wrinkled hands and give them a more youthful look.

As a practicing plastic surgeon, I look forward to the day when age comes into its own as a symbol of *meaningful maturity*, not dread and senescence. That will be the day when we come to fully realize that life is BEING, ENJOYING, and not to be measured by birthdays alone. That will be the day when our frenetic concern with youth has turned into the realities of not only a longer life, but a better one.

Meanwhile, in our justified enthusiasm for what the injection method can do, let us not jump to conclusions about its effect on the whole field of plastic surgery. Just as Univac has not completely replaced the human factor, the padding is an adjunct to the field, but by no means a complete replacement.

For some, if used in time in small delicate injections, it can indeed be a major answer. For others, it can give new meaning to necessary surgery when combined with it. When there is too much sag or hanging skin, there will remain many cases where the scalpel, together with injection therapy, is the answer. Large injections are not the answer, nor is it effective for breast enlargement—the simple surgical approach being best.

"Cleopatra's Needle" has given us a development such as, say, the self-starter was to the automobile. That replaced the crank, but not the machine itself. The framework of plastic surgery remains as the body, or machine, improved but not replaced.

Banish Wrinkles in a Wink!

CHAPTER TWENTY-FOUR

Beauty begins with a flawless skin. If you treat your own skin, be sure you select the correct products. Unjudicious selection of beauty aids can do more harm than good. Study your skin. What are its flaws? Are there rough, reddish areas and little blood vessels apparent around the edges of the nose and mouth? If so, this is a sure sign that you have exposed your face to too much sun and wind. Therefore, a general treatment for the circulation is indicated. However, this does *not* exclude local treatments, too. Applications of products made of sea salts are advised for decongesting the skin and preventing further complications. Medical treatments such as carbonic snow, or jet sprays are also beneficial. Be very careful not to irritate your skin if it is in bad condition. Do not wash it in water which is too hot or too cold. Use only the mildest of soaps.

Are there little wrinkles around your eyes? Then use products with an absorbable base which contain vitamin rich amino acids. These are excellent for smoothing away those skin wrinkles. Skins that are oily, pimply or subject

221

to blackheads usually resist sun damage, but unfortunately they don't become any more attractive because of it. Such skins need frequent applications of aromatic lotions which are antiseptic and astringent. If the condition is particularly bad, special medical care is advised. (One treatment which is wonderful for this is the use of pure ozone.)

Whatever your skin troubles, there are modern techniques which are excellent means of defense against the aging appearance of the skin. Aesthetic surgery can do wonders in rejuvenation by tightening the lax skin of the face, thus restoring a youthful smoothness. There is another method which requires no surgery. This is *dermabrasion*.

Dermabrasion, as practiced by the specialists, consists of applications of a spinning diamond wheel which removes a layer of the epidermis. Since the skin conditions and qualities differ from person to person, each subject must be treated individually. The specialists of this method of rejuvenating the skin have made profound studies of the many skin types and vary their treatments accordingly.

The surface is skimmed off. Under this tired surface lies new, smooth, unblemished skin that will soon replace the old skin. Once the new skin is exposed, however, it *must* be cared for because it is very delicate.

For the ravages of age—droopy, excess skin—the simplest process is the Mini Face Lift which takes only minutes to do. A few days later, the stitches are removed. The result is immediate! The whole procedure is as simple as going to a beauty parlor. Often this is done in conjunction with an injection or two of the Cleopatra's Needle to plump out the sunken lines and hollows of the face which often precede the droopy face.

The process of aging usually becomes visible when a woman reaches twenty-six or twenty-seven, when bags begin to appear under the eyes. As a woman gets older she acquires puffy areas and loose skin on her face. If these are attended to early enough, one only requires a minor eye lift in which the excess skin and puffs are removed. The operation, which takes only minutes, is very satisfying in terms of results achieved. In this operation, tiny slits are made and the excess skin removed. Within three days the area is almost devoid of all signs of any surgery. It is the fastest healing of all operations and leaves no trace of the fact that any work has ever been done.

As a woman ages, her cheeks tend to droop around the eye area. At twenty-nine or thirty deep lines or grooves usually appear between the nose and the mouth. In this instance, the Cleopatra's Needle technique works on eliminating these facial grooves. Here, too, the Mini Face Lift might be recommended. The surgery is performed *inside* the hairline area of the temple, thereby restoring the face to its previous youthful look. In addition, an advantage of the Mini Face Lift is that all traces of the operation are hidden within the hairline without having to have the hair shaved. No one—but the lady in question—need ever know she's had this type of operation.

If a woman allows herself to reach her late forties, or fifties or even her sixties without taking advantage of the Cleopatra's Needle technique or a minor eye lift or a Mini Face Lift, then a major face lift may be in order. If a major face lift is required this, too, is a relatively uncomplicated procedure from the patient's point of view. A major face lift requires less than an hour of surgery and is done around and behind the ears. In this operation the excess skin from the neck and face is smoothed upward and removed requiring only a minimum of tiny stitches which are removed within seven or ten days.

All of the operations and facial improvements I've mentioned are done with a local anesthetic and with the patient in a sitting up position. No hospitalization is required. A patient comes in the morning and leaves that same morning under her own power. Unlike the arduous procedure of years ago, in which several days or even a week's hospitalization was advocated during which the patient was heavily bandaged, I believe in allowing the patient to get up immediately and to move around and resume her normal way of life. Not only does the patient feel better but the results are much more natural physically, as well as more mentally beneficial.

The sooner you become familiar with these modern day "cosmetic miracles," the quicker you will achieve lasting **beauty!**

To Wig or not to Wig? What a Question!

CHAPTER TWENTY-FIVE

Hair care is essential when it comes to considering overall beauty. A mane of healthy, lustrous hair is a must. Fortunately, today's women are in a better position to have lovely hair than even the titled ladies of yesterday. The solution to hair problems can be found in one little word—WIG.

Since the advent of the wig, fall, and wiglet cult in America, more women have saved more time and looked far better than ever before. No longer is it necessary to spend countless hours at the beauty shop . . . nor is it compulsory for milady to go to sleep all done up in rollers, looking like the left tackle from some professional football team. Now a woman can be well-groomed every hour of her life—and at a surprisingly low cost.

Several words of caution are in order. First, if it is at all possible do NOT economize on your basic wig. While it is certainly not necessary to spend hundreds of dollars on a hairpiece, it is also unwise to buy an inexpensive one—say in the twenty to fifty dollar range. There certainly are many wigs on the market for this price, wigs which look glorious in the store windows and dreadful after you've worn them a few times. Rather than buy a wig which will NOT really do the job, you're better off to save for a good one and make do with a wiglet until such time as you can afford a nice, substantial bit of hair.

The trouble with the cheaper wigs is that they are made of a synthetic fiber which does not hold up under heavy duty. What is worse, such wigs begin to look fake after the original luster is gone, and then you have a bunch of obviously synthetic hair on your hands—or head—as the case may be.

Do not misunderstand. There are some very nice falls—single hanks of hair which are used to add to already long hair, to braid, to make a bun, to act as an accessory to one's own hair. These falls *do* come moderately priced, and even the less expensive ones—when blended skillfully with your own hair—can serve your purpose nicely. But for the full wig, economizing isn't wise.

Because wig selection is such a personal matter, we shall skip to a more basic point—namely THE CARE AND HANDLING OF YOUR WIG. This is a very important topic for the potential wig owner who wants to "Play the Beauty Game." Like a car, a wig must be kept up. Many woman are scared of buying wigs because they panic at the anticipation of huge beauty shop bills to set, shampoo and style the wig after purchase. While it is true that a wig *should* be professionally styled at the time of purchase, it is NOT true that you have to be a slave to a beauty salon constantly thereafter.

How to Handle Your Wig at Home

1. Any woman who can roll her own hair can now set

and style her own wig right at home. All it takes is a bit of practice until you have enough confidence in your ability to handle this new beauty aid.

2. Along with your wig purchase buy an inexpensive styrofoam form to hold your hairpiece. To hold the wig in place, you will need either long hatpins or T-pins which are readily available wherever wigs are sold. Always pin the wig to the form, first at the front comb spot, then use another pin to anchor the back down, and, if necessary, use one pin on each side.

3. When you are working with the wig on the form, it is possible to handle it without any other aids. However, there is an inexpensive vacuum-type holder on the market which acts like a suction cup and sticks to the table firmly anchoring the form so it will not move while you go about your wig grooming.

4. Once your wig is firmly attached to the form, and you have placed it so that it is easy to work with, you are ready to brush or comb your wig just as though it were the hair growing on your head. If you want to keep the same style in which the wig was orginally, then comb and brush it in sections, keeping the styling the same and following the original set.

If you wish to restyle the wig, first brush and comb the hair back and down—just as you do your own hair. If the wig previously has been teased, don't lose patience. It is easy to untangle the hairs if you go slowly, keeping one hand firmly at the base of the wig and untangling small sections at a time with your fingers and a brush.

Give the wig a good brushing. Be sure to remove all the dust, hair spray and general soil which might have accumulated through wear. If you brush and comb your wig frequently, it won't need so many washings.

5. A good wig is originally made of strong, young, healthy hair, hair that takes a good curl and keeps one. It stands to reason that wig hair, which is not subjected to normal wear and tear such as your own hair is, stays better longer. You don't sleep in it. No body oil or perspiration interferes with the set—therefore a good wig is like a good gem—hardy and beautiful.

6. In setting your wig it is essential that you DO NOT use clips or curlers with fold-over closures, or bobby pins. Wire rollers in various sizes are the easiest tools with which to work. NOTE: Do NOT use wire rollers with brushes inside as they prevent your getting a nice smooth curl.

7. Now, divide the hair into small sections, planning where each curl will go just the same way as you do when you set your own hair. Start at the ends and roll the hair around the roller, then pin it into the styrofoam form with a hat pin or the T-pins.

8. For bangs or other straight sections just comb into place. If necessary, turn the ends to one side and hold fast with a thin "invisible-type" hairpin.

9. If it is easier for you to work with dry hair, just proceed to roll the entire wig and then spray lightly with plain water. (Fill any bottle and use an atomizer top to add the water, making sure not to douse the wig too much.) Remember, it is neither necessary nor wise to over-do the amount of water used. Just a slight spray is adequate to set the hair nicely. Also, do NOT use hair wave lotions or gels—they are unnecessary and will not leave the hair looking as lovely or natural as a plain water set will.

10. If you are in a rush for your wig, it may be dried with any regular home hair dryer. However, if you have

more time, place the styrofoam form under a table lamp for a while, the heat of the bulb will dry it nicely.

11. The comb-out of your wig is as easy as a regular comb out of natural hair. First, pull out the pins which have been anchoring the wig. Carefully remove the rollers and place the wig on your head. Secure it with bobby pins under the band and at each side to assure that it is firmly in place. When the wig is secure, comb through as though it were your own hair, teasing, brushing, smoothing down as usual.

NOTE: With a wiglet (purchased to match your own hair) skillfully blend the wig hair into your own so no one but you will be able to tell where wig begins and you leave off.

12. A big problem is in wig cleaning. Today, there are some good wig cleaners for sale at any drug store, beauty salon, or department store notions' section. Select a good dry cleaner and follow the directions on the label carefully.

13. However, *you may shampoo your wig at home if you are careful.* Buy a good shampoo (your beauty operator will tell you the right type of shampoo to buy for your particular wig.) Follow package directions for shampooing. In general, please note that a wig MUST NEVER BE RUBBED EXCESSIVELY OR MANIPULATED WHILE IT IS IN THE SHAMPOO SOLUTION OR UNDER THE WATER. Usually fifteen to twenty minutes of soaking will clean a wig thoroughly. Let the water run through the wig gently. No excessive force or pressure is needed. After all, your wig does NOT have an oily scalp or excessive dandruff to clean. Then, holding the hairpiece by the comb inside the band, attach the comb over your wash basin or tub and allow it to drip-dry until all the moisture has dripped through. Then replace the wig

on its form, comb, set and style as usual. NOTE: Try as little teasing as possible—a wig bulks up your own hairstyle anyway. Teasing excessively is hard on a wig and should be done with moderation. Other than this, use your wig happily without fear of hurting it. You will find it is able to withstand more than your own natural hair for longer periods of time without getting messy looking.

When it comes to "Milady's Crowning Glory," the judicious purchase and use of falls, wiglets and full wigs is one of the quickest roads to beauty. You can and should be daring, tempestuous, seductive—a lovely wig goes a long way toward helping you accomplish your goals!

The Shampoo

If your hair is extremely dry, try giving yourself a hot oil treatment before beginning your shampoo. Warm some olive oil and saturate wads of absorbent cotton with it. Apply it all over your scalp. Place a heating cap or hot towel on your head for twenty minutes.

Then wet your entire head with warm—not hot—water. Distribute the shampoo evenly on your scalp. Rub the shampoo in either with your fingers or with a rubber scalp brush (An old toothbrush is good for rubbing along the hairline.) Rinse your hair. Repeat the process once more for dry hair.

Wrap your head turban-style in a towel, blotting the water. If your hair has a tendency to break, don't rub it dry.

A few drops of bluing in the final rinse water will enhance the sheen of gray hair. A tablespoon of vinegar or lemon juice in a quart of water is an excellent final rinse for dry hair. Or, you may prefer a cream rinse.

Yours may be the kind of hair that requires a special shampoo. If your hair has been lightened, toned or tinted, it needs a special shampoo that conditions as it cleans. If your hair is oily, you'll need a deep-cleaning shampoo that has no extra oils. If your hair is dry, you should try a shampoo that contains emollients. If your hair tends to be limp, a shampoo that contains protein compounds may add body.

A wide range of special shampoos for special effects are available today, including color shampoos that brighten your natural shade.

How to Color-Test Your Hair

One out of every two women in the United States does something about the color of her hair. If she doesn't actually dye it, she at least "color rinses" it.

If you are thinking about changing your hair color, you needn't take an irrevocable step. You can try out a temporary color in the privacy of your own home.

Before using one of the new, and effective, temporary color products, test the product on a small patch of your scalp. If you have an allergic reaction, the product is not for you. (Follow directions included with the product.)

You can experiment with new color via a color rinse that deposits color on the outside of the hair shaft and can be removed immediately through shampooing.

You might try a shampoo tint that will accentuate one of the natural colors of your hair.

If you're almost, but not quite, convinced that you want a permanent color change, try one of the semi-permanent rinses. These don't rub off and they last for several weeks.

Color rinses are particularly effective for hair that is beginning to fade.

You can test these color rinses safely by taking the patch test and following the directions provided by the manufacturer. Dyes, however, require the hand of the professional.

Before you make a final decision on changing your hair color permanently, consider all the extra care your hair will require. Dyes *do* cause dryness. You will need to pay more attention to your hair and scalp to avoid this condition. Additional visits to the hairdresser will be necessary. If you should change your mind after taking that final step, you'll have to suffer through a "growing back" period.

Of course, today's woman has another alternative—the wig!

Permanents

If your hair is coarse, a machine wave or a wave that uses chemically treated pads will probably be best for you. If you hair is fine, your hairdresser will probably suggest a cold wave.

Before listing the benefits of a permanent, here are a few words of caution:

1. Don't get a permanent within three or four months of your last one.

2. Don't get a permanent within three or four months of dying or bleaching your hair.

3. Don't get a permanent if your scalp has any cuts, scratches or other irritations.

4. Don't get a permanent until one strand of you hair has successfully passed a "patch test" of the waving solution.

The important thing to be sure of is that your permanent wave is customized especially for you—from the haircut, to the type and size of roller that is to be used, to the strength of the solution to be used.

After you have your permanent, be sure to give your

hair the same careful attention you would give it if it were waveless.

Selecting A Hair-Style

Your hair-style should glamorize the shape of your face. It should, at the same time, draw attention away from any physical shortcomings you may have. If you are too short or too tall, the right hair-style can give a counteracting illusion. The proper hair-style can cleverly conceal unsightly ears. It can even detract from a nose that is too long.

The first step to take in trying to select a flattering hair-style is a step toward your mirror. Study your face carefully, noting which features you would like most to emphasize, or to camouflage. First, look at your nose. If it's too long or too large, keep curls and waves set back high for balance. Be sure curls and waves are large—small ones will merely emphasize the size of the nose. Never part your hair in the middle. If your nose is too short or too small, bring bangs and curls below your hairline. A feathercut will probably help. Avoid upsweeps.

How about your chin? If it recedes, you can strengthen its appearance by bringing your side hair forward in curls below the ears. If it juts out, wear your hair full and high at the top and brushed back from the hairline at the sides. If it is a double-chin, the upsweep is for you.

Now, how's your forehead? If your forehead is high, you can cover part of it with a partial wave or with bangs or a fluff. If it is low, you can heighten it with an off-the-face sweep. If you must have bangs, keep them short.

Sun Fun

CHAPTER TWENTY-SEVEN

Most women think they look better with a glowing tan.
Often looks are deceptive. While a bronzed complexion
appears most alluring, it *can* be harmful. If you vacation
at a seaside resort or any area where exposure to the sun is
part of your daily ritual there are some important Do's
and Don'ts.

First: The time of the sunbath. During the first few
days of your holiday do not expose youself to the sun's rays
right after lunch for this is when the sun's intensity is
greatest. The rule should be: sun bathe before eleven and
after three o'clock until the dermal tolerance is built up.

Second: The duration of a sunbath. Generally, this
depends upon your individual tolerance, your type of skin
and your organic reactions. Don't ignore any of these factors. If you are a city dweller and spend most of your time
indoors for eleven months of the year, don't try to get a
tan in one fell swoop. Follow a progressive exposure program. Start with the body portions which are most resist-
ant to the effects of the sun's rays. Ten minutes is sufficient for a beginner. During those ten minutes you should
not stay in one position. Turn frequently.

Since the sun's rays are not constant, turn with the sun, in order to find the ideal position. As the shadow moves, turn your body also, always keeping it at a right angle to the shadow. Eventually you will be able to increase your ten minute exposures to thirty or forty-five minutes, but even then you should continue to turn the body often. Keep your head covered and your eyes protected with sunglasses at all times. If your association with the sun is already established then, of course, the rules are less strict. Your own intelligence is the only thing to guide you. Use it.

You will get a good tan, without danger, if you alternate sunbathing with dips in the ocean and if you protect your skin with frequent and plentiful applications of sun oils or creams with filtrant properties.

Don't attempt to get tanned while taking a long nap on the beach. Above all, get out of the sun immediately if you feel the slightest bit feverish. This is an indication of sunstroke. If unfortunately you should get an excessive case of sunburn, regard it in the same manner as any other type of burn. *Treat it at once.* If the case is serious, it may require the attention of a doctor or even hospitalization. Incidentally, one can get sunburned easiest in a standing position because the salty perspiration drips on the body and, where it collects, the skin burns. When you are lying down the perspiration is more-or-less evenly distributed over the body and dries up. However, standing up, or lying down, dry yourself frequently with a towel.

Third: Never go out into the sun without taking along a protective covering. The sun can turn your face into a wrinkled prune. Too much sun can trigger an organic reaction. The results can be dangerous both aesthetically and health-wise because the internal upset can in turn cause: thickened cracked skin, spots, pimples, and even skin pigmentation and acne.

Fourth: Remember, if moderation and common sense are applied, sunbathing can benefit your health, your beauty and your peace of mind.

Winter Sun

Devout sun worshippers are as eager to tan in the wintertime as they are during the summer months. However, sun devotees who go in for winter sports such as skiing should understand that the reflection of sun rays on snow and ice can be far more dangerous than the direct rays of a summer sun if protective measures are not taken. The dangers are not limited to the aesthetic properties, but also bear upon the entire system. Sun rays penetrate deep into the body. Any over-exposure to the ultraviolet rays will cause a drying out of the skin glands and the skin, in self-defense, becomes tough and thick. Then, too, there are the surface reactions such as wrinkling, freckling, red and painful burns which over a prolonged period can cause permanent damage and eventually undermine one's general health. While it is true that some people have more resistance than others, depending on whether they are accustomed to out-of-doors living and continual exposure to the sun, still sunstroke, headaches and eye troubles are not uncommon even to those hardy souls who are used to the conditions.

The ultra-violet rays of the sun cause erythema as well as the peeling of the outer layers of skin. These are not the rays that make the skin turn brown, because they do not penetrate. The infra-red rays are the ones that cause the skin to tan, and they are less harmful than the others even though they do penetrate the epidermis.

Exposure to the sun in high altitudes should be approached with the same precautions that one would observe at the seashore in the hot summer months. In fact, precautions are even more vital since the sun in high alti-

tudes is very rich in ultra-violet rays. Therefore tanning
sessions should be progressive and the skin defended with
a coating of oil or cream that is both filtrant and protective. Applications of whatever product is used should be
repeated frequently because the protective film is quickly
absorbed by the skin. Removal of the product should be
used since it may contain harmful chemical properties
which could have adverse effects on the skin after exposure
to the sun.

Caution: Protect your eyes as they are very susceptible
to the effects of sunlight. Ocular congestion, caused by the
ultra-violet rays of mountain sunshine, is just one of the
risks to be faced if the eyes are not protected. Equally possible are: conjunctivitis, sunburned retina, and the formation of wrinkles around the eyes. Avoidance of these perils
is simple: Always wear sun glasses. Sun glasses with dark
brown or gray lenses should be worn when the sun is
bright, yellow lenses when the sky is overcast. Don't be
fooled into thinking that just because there are clouds
hiding the sun its rays are not filtering through.

During the day in the snow, always protect your skin
with a lotion which will keep it from drying out. Wear no
make-up except an oily lipstick, and a bit of hydrant
creme on the eyelids. For evening you can of course apply
your usual cosmetics. Have your hair protected when
out-of-doors and give it a thorough, but gentle brushing
when you come indoors. Massaging your feet, hands and
legs with vitaminized nourishing cream will lessen the pos-
sibility of chapping. You can protect your hands and feet
from becoming wet by wearing silk gloves and hose underneath your woolen stockings and mittens. Your shoes
should be absolutely waterproof. It would be a good idea
if your mittens were likewise.

Also, a diet in which there is a sufficiency of calcium and
vitamins, particularly vitamin C, not only helps to keep

the body in good state, but also aids in the tanning process.

By following the foregoing suggestions your vacation in the winter sun can be beneficial to your health and beauty.

Summertime Tips

Hot, humid weather can take a toll in physical discomfort if you over-exercise or are over-exposed to the sun, especially if you are not in good condition. You CAN condition yourself for summer exercise and sun-bathing and learn to live with hot weather. The older you are and the more sedentary your winter life, the more planning is required for gradual conditioning. This does not mean you should not excercise in the summer. Exercise can help condition the body to hot weather so that your cooling mechanisms function better making you more comfortable. However, a few words of caution are in order.

A. Do not exercise in the midday heat or after a heavy meal.

B. Work or play at a pace that does not overtire you. Short rests (ten minutes out of each hour) are more beneficial than a few long ones.

C. Engage in sports BEFORE sun-bathing if you wish to be at your best. Sun-bathing is enervating and lowers performance.

D. More sleep is needed with more exercise. Do not try to stay up late and play hard all day.

Although no major changes in diet are necessary in the summer, and hot meals do not have to be avoided, many people prefer cold dishes and iced drinks. However, fewer calories are needed in summer so you can eat sparingly and keep fat intake down. It is not true that the more you drink in hot weather, the more you perspire. Replacing body fluids lost in sweat is important to summer health, especially fluids lost through exercise. Too much ice water drunk at a gulp can cause stomach cramps, but, if the water is not iced, drink to your thirst. Any excess is eliminated through the kidneys, not through perspiration. Those who drink alcoholic beverages in warm weather should do so cautiously. Their sudden effect can make you ill or, at least, make you feel warmer. You also sweat more which can add to your discomfort.

Your body's supply of salt is diminished through sweating, especially during exercise before you have become adjusted to summer heat. For most people, salt is replaced by a normal diet. For those who are active and perspire a lot, an extra shake or two of salt on food will be adequate to replenish the supply. Lack of salt and depletion of body fluids through perspiration coupled with hot, humid weather can cause heat exhaustion.

Because lightweight, light-colored clothing is porous, it can keep you cooler. The body surface is cooled by evaporation of sweat, a function that is retarded by close-fitting or tightly-woven clothing. Hats are advisable if you are in the sun. Hats which allow air circulation, such as straw or helmet-types suspended from an inner band, are most beneficial. During strenuous play or work in hot weather, letting a blouse or shirttail hang out at the waist and leaving collars open helps cool by ventilation. Keeping skin and clothes clean helps evaporation and promotes cooling.

Massage:
Rub-a-Dub-Dub

*In the realm of beauty aids massaging can occupy a decid-*edly important place. Although a lot has been written about massaging, many false notions have been pro-pounded. While massages have long been known to be a means of activating the distribution of blood properties and lymph in the skin, there is still much to be learned about their over-all effects upon the body. The use of mas-sage is as old as recorded time. In one ancient tomb we find massaging described as "the method with which women can maintain their figures and the splendor of their skins".

We do know that massaging is certainly the safest means of stimulating the physiological functions and maintaining the normality of the skin. Because of this it is one of the best methods of beautifying the face, the neck and the bust. Certain massage procedures can facilitate the func-tions of the sebaceous glands and at the same time rid the skin of blackheads and other subsurface accumulations which give it a granular appearance. Then, too, the manipulations help to tone up the skin and improve the nourishment of the muscles, which, in turn, helps them to retain, or regain, their vigor and functioning powers.

Massaging is an art which requires expert knowledge in order to make beneficial readjustments of the functioning of the vast nerve network underlying the skin layers. It is this nerve network that causes our sensatory reaction to external conditions. For instance, consider the "common headache"—nothing can diminish pleasure or interest in work more than a headache. However, relief usually can be brought about through a light massaging of the forehead and the temples in order to ease the tensions on the nerves and the muscles. This massaging has a two-fold benefit in that it also helps to smooth out those wrinkles, euphemistically called "lines of expression".

Modern science has delved into the benefits derived from various massage techniques and has found that among other things, they bring about a decongesting of the fluid in the body's connective tissues. In addition, the sustenance of the body tissues is augmented by the acceleration of the molecular distribution of energy properties.

Various massage manipulations can not only create a general feeling of well being—but also can give visible results. The latter is especially noted when massage is employed for cosmetic reasons, which is to say, for beautifying the face and body. Here, however, we must hasten to add that caution is the keyword. The skin of the face may be compared to a harp with many cords (the nerve network) which often needs tuning in order to be beautiful and in best working condition. But only someone who is familiar with the instrument can keep it in tune. So, too, massaging can be beneficial if done by a specialist who understands the structure of the delicate skin covering of the face.

Massages differ according to desired results:

For the most part a circulatory massage motion is used as a means of unclogging the surface tissues. To be done properly the hands should move gently over the face and the neck in a centripetal motion in order to stimulate the flow of blood toward the heart. The massage movements may be slow or rapid depending upon the desired results. If the movements are light they will soothe and calm. If more force is applied it will act to decontract the muscles and activate the ciruclation.

Kneading, pinching, and pummeling are techniques used to prevent the skin and muscles from becoming slack. These manipulations tone up the muscles by stimulating their nourishment intake which in turn increases the traction faculties of the muscle fibers. Muscular atrophy or flaccidity are treated with these techniques.

Rhythmic, quick tappings are used as shock stimulants for increasing the circulation through the treated regions and to heighten the nourishment intake of the tissues. It also decontracts and tones the muscles. There are various tapping methods: with the open hand, or the tips of the fingers, and even mechanical appliances which give vibratory tapping.

All of the above mentioned massage techniques are only parts of a series. Any amelioration of a body condition can only be achieved through a routine of the complete series.

Turning to the mechanical means of massaging we find that there are machines which create varying vibrations that give excellent results. These mechanical massages are, in some ways, better than the manual ones for regenerating and stimulating the skin tissues. The constancy of vibrations tends to quicken the results and the vibratory waves help to re-establish the elasticity of the tissues. Herein may lie the key to the secret of rejuvenation, because, as we all know, the lack of circulation in the body tissues is directly connected with the aging processes.

It is evident that in order to be effective any mechanical massage should be administered by a qualified technician. However, this does not completely exclude self-massaging techniques. The primary drawback in applying a mechanical vibrator to one's own face is the general lack of knowledge of the anatomical structure of the face. Even so, one can, by observing certain rules, decontract the facial muscles and smooth out wrinkles with the use of a massage apparatus.

Here is what you can do yourself:

With hands flat and pressed lightly on the forehead, stroke towards the hair.

To smooth out crows-feet, work from the temples and follow the outlines of the face.

When working on the eyelids and around the eyes, use light pressing movements as this will prevent the formation of pouches and ease any feelings of tiredness of the eyes.

The neck: the hand should be firmly placed on the neck area to be treated and a stroking movement used.

Stand up to Beauty: Your Feet, Hands, Eyes & Ears

Most probably during your lifetime you will walk around 65,000 miles. To do that and still keep smiling, you need healthy feet. Why worry? Because tired feet affect facial beauty.

Since your feet bear your weight, maintain your balance, and get you from place to place, they deserve to be given the proper care. One of the most common abuses of the feet is wearing shoes selected for *style* rather than comfort, causing ingrown toenails, corns, bunions and even bone deformation. In fact, these conditions can be aggravated to a point where the only corrective measure is an operation. Shoe heels can be high for elegant occasions, but shoes made for walking, or standing on for long periods at a time, should be half-heels or very low ones. Sandals and ballet slippers should get part-time wear since they offer little support for the foot.

Also, massage your feet with special creams and lotions, keep your toenails trimmed properly, and visit a podiatrist periodically. Your feet will feel better, and serve you better.

Foot Exercises

A. Stand with your feet about five inches apart. Slowly lift your heels until you are balancing on the balls of your feet and on your toes. Descend extremely slowly.

B. Walking in your bare feet around a room, walking on the edges of your feet, first on the outside edge and then inside. Stop occasionally to pick up a pencil from the floor with your toes.

C. Stand on the floor. Rock back and forth, from toes to heels and then from one side of the foot to the other.

D. Sit on a chair. Extend your feet before you. Point the toes forward as far as possible, then point them up and back toward you as far as possible. Repeat ten times.

Pedicure

1. Wash and dry your feet carefully (or clean them with the lotion you usually use for cleaning your face).

2. Trim the nails. In order to do a good job of nail-trimming you need a pair of strong scissors or a nail clipper. The end of the nail should be carefully smoothed off so it will not tear your stockings.

3. Remove the excess cuticle with a small pair of cuticle scissors, or with the cuticle oil used for manicure. If you use a cuticle oil, be sure to wash it off before proceeding with the pedicure.

4. Now you are ready for creaming and massaging. Around the cuticle and nails place a small quantity of cold cream or petroleum jelly (vaseline). Allow this to soak in

while you cover the rest of your foot with a thin layer of cream—almost any cream you may happen to have will answer for this purpose. Massage thoroughly. There is no special technique required for this purpose; simply manipulate and massage all parts of the foot.

5. Remove the cream with facial tissue.

6. Apply nail polish if you desire, using the same polish and technique you ordinarily use on your fingernails.

7. Apply toilet water or scented talcum, if you like.

Hand Care

Your hands have much to say about you, about the way you feel and the way you think. They express your personality. Hands can say you are young by their firmness and smoothness. They can say that you are healthy and care for yourself by their delicate softness. They can say that you are graceful by the way they move. They can express your beauty *if they are beautiful.*

Your hands need special attention. They should be soft, smooth and topped off with well-kept fingernails. These qualities are the result of daily care.

Your hands are apt to be dryer than your face and the rest of your body because the skin on your hands has fewer oil cells than the rest of you does. Therefore, hands do need special care. They need a soap rich in fat . . . they need protective covering . . . they need a special routine to replace lost moisture.

Your nails need calcium, Vitamin B and proteins for health. If these elements are missing in the body, your health suffers. Therefore, your nails serve as a sign of health deficiencies. Proper diet and vitamin-intake, plus care, can enhance the shiny transparency and the smooth surface of the nails.

There are many household and professional tasks that

can impair the beauty of hands, especially if the hands come in contact with irritating products such as detergents which cause excessive dryness. In dishwashing, there is another enemy along with detergents.

Hot Water

For good and proper hand care, do *not* use very hot water. When washing more than a few dishes at a time, use a pair of rubber gloves. Finally, don't neglect to pamper your hands with one of the many hand lotions which are on the market.

Hand Blemishes

Any stubborn discoloration should be examined by a physician. The same is true of warts. Never try to deal with such blemishes yourself. If there are simple brown spots or red scales on your hands, apply a product which will remove the superficial exfoliation of the skin. Massage frequently with a bleaching lotion, or more simply with the juice of a lemon.

You can easily take care of simple callouses at home. Soap up the callous and rub it using a gentle circular motion with a slightly-dampened pumice stone. If the callouses persist, see a physician.

Sweaty Hands

Nothing is more unpleasant than clasping a sweaty hand. The condition, which may be due to nervousness or hypertension, requires special medical treatments. At the same time, the condition should be treated with alum baths and massages with powders containing drying agents. Deodorants should also be employed. Normally, a hand should not be dry as parchment—neither should it be damp as a sponge.

Chapped Hands

The first thing needed to treat chapped hands is a pair of clean white gloves. Massage your hands with a rich hand cream, getting it into every pore. Apply a thick coat of cream and slip on the gloves—preferably an oversize pair. Repeat several times a day. If you must be before the public during the day, wear the gloves only at night, but replenish cream frequently during the day.

Brittle Nails

A hot oil treatment is excellent for brittle nails that split or break easily. Another important step is to remove nail polish and to keep it off for several days during the first series of treatments. Once the situation is under control, select one night a week that it is possible for you to be without nail polish. Remove the polish, take the treatment and sleep sans nail polish.

For the treatment, heat a portion of vegetable oil and soak your fingertips for twenty minutes. Wipe the fingers dry with absorbent cotton. Be sure to leave a coating of oil on your nails. During the first series of treatments, dab a bit of oil on your nails as often as possible during the day.

After the condition has improved, an occasional oil treatment should do. You might also apply white iodine once a week to your polish-free nails to make them stronger. Be sure your manicure products have an oily base. Nail polish remover can make your nails brittle unless it is of the oily variety.

Diet plays an important part in fingernail strength. Be sure that you are consuming sufficient protein. The "B for Beauty" vitamin-intake is also important. Ask your physician about the advisability of increasing your calcium intake via calcium tablets, at least until your nails grow harder.

Give Your Hands A Beauty Bath

Never use hot water to wash your hands—absolutely never! Use lukewarm water in a basin and pure soap for the bath. If your hands tend to be oily, use a handbrush. Otherwise, use a wash cloth.

Dip your hands into the bath and rub the soap vigorously to make suds. Massage the suds into your hands with a washcloth or brush. Be sure to get under your nails and around your cuticles.

Use your pumice stone while your water is still soapy.

When rinsing, use only lukewarm water. Remove every bit of soap. As you dry your hands, press back your cuticles, gently.

Massage a small amount of hand cream or lotion into your hands until it has all been absorbed.

When polish is dry, apply a clear top coat to finish manicure. Cover entire nail surface and bring over the tip edge, letting the top coat flow under the nail tip. This seals the polish, prevents chipping.

For healthier, stronger nails, massage nail cream into base of nails and around cuticles every night. Nail cream strengthens the matrix or growing portion of nail that lies under the skin at base of nail. It helps prevent nail peeling and splitting. But it must be used faithfully for a period of time before a marked difference will be noted.

If polish becomes worn or chipped between manicures, remove it if you don't have time for repairs. Soft, weak nails will not hold polish as long as healthy ones. Newest fashion colors are lighter and softer. Polish should match or harmonize with lipstick.

Hand Exercises

Try these four exercises daily to help your circulation, and to keep your hands and fingers slender and supple.

1. Stand with your feet twelve inches apart. Extend your arms to the side, then raise them high above your head. Holding your hands stiff, swing your arms in windmill motions. Repeat ten times.

2. Sit at a table. Rest your arms on the elbows. Clench your hands together into two tight fists. Open each fist, spreading each finger out as far as possible, bending the fingers as far backward as possible—to form two hand fans. Repeat seven times.

3. Stand with your feet about twelve inches apart. Arms at your sides. Keeping elbows at waist level, raise hands to your shoulders. Shake your hands loosely from your wrists in a circular motion. Continue for one minute.

4. From elbow to wrist, knead your arms with your fingertips—first one arm and then the other. Then, taking one hand in the other, place the thumb of the second hand in the palm of the first and the four fingers of the second on the back of the first. Knead gently, being sure to work on all muscles and knuckles. With the same motion, massage each finger, working up to the tip. Repeat with the other hand.

White hands: If your hands are swollen and stiff it may be due to poor circulation, and this should be checked into. Spraying your hands several times a day with alternated hot and cold water, carrying your hands high, and swinging your arms in windmill motions will help to activate the circulation. If there are brown spots or red scales on your hands, apply a product which will remove the superficial exfoliation of the skin. Massage frequently with a bleaching lotion or, more simply, with the juice of a le·.1on. Or, for a do-it-yourself remedy: Prick a vitamin E Capsule and apply oil to spots. Continue for several months until spots fade.

Flexible hands: We must once again stress the importance of physical culture because there is simply no means of making the wrist and fingers supple other than constant and appropriate exercises. If you play the piano it is an excellent means of keeping your fingers and hands agile; however, you can get the same exercises on a table. Another good hand limbering exercise is to roll a marble between the fingers or, clasping a ball, rotate the hand from the wrist.

Expressive hands: Hands can sometimes express sentiments more charmingly than words. It requires practice to learn to do this properly. Don't be afraid to use your hands when speaking, but *don't* use them too much. There is a happy medium that can enhance your personality.

Stylish hands: Your nails should be kept neatly trimmed and polished. If your nails have a tendency to be fragile and break easily it may be an indication of a physical malajustment. In addition to correcting any physical deficiency—if such exists—you should also give your nails special treatments with revitalizing products to help them become more firm. Give the nails an almond shape when filing them with a soft emery, then soften the cuticle with a suitable cream or oil and push it back with an orange stick. Don't cut away the dead skin. Instead, use a cuticle remover and buffer for this. When the nails are well cleaned and shaped they are ready to be polished. Select a color that matches your lipstick. After applying a coating of nail base protector give the nails two coatings of polish. Over this apply a protector to keep the polish from chipping. A professional manicurist can do a better and longer lasting job for you, but with a little time and effort you can keep your own nails neat and attractive in between professional manicures.

Hand Tips—The Manicure

1. Remove old polish with oily polish remover.

2. With a drop of a cuticle softener, massage nails. Gently push back cuticle with an orange stick. (It is unwise to cut the cuticle, as this causes hangnails.) If you have a hangnail, clip the rough, loosened cuticle, then leave it alone. Regular use of a cuticle softener will prevent further development of hangnails.

3. Wash and dry nails thoroughly. Clean, dry nails hold nail polish much longer.

4. Shape nails into ovals with emery board. Do not file nails away at the corners because this seriously weakens nails and speeds breakage. File in one direction only.

5. Cover entire surface of your nail with a base coat. Bring brush clear to the tip of the nail for better wear. A base coat forms a pliant, smooth film over the nail. Polish will not last if applied over a rough, uneven surface.

6. Apply two coats of polish with firm, deliberate strokes. Allow the first coat to dry before applying the second coat.

7. To delay chipping, remove a hairsbreadth of polish around the tip of each nail with a bit of cotton and polish remover. This professional trick helps prolong the life of your polish, makes manicures last. (Caution: Don't smear fresh polish with wet cotton.)

8. When your polish is dry, apply a clear top coat to finish manicure. Cover entire nail surface and bring over the tip edge, letting the top coat flow under the nail tip. This seals the polish, prevents chipping.

9. For healthier nails massage nail cream into base of nails and around cuticles every night. Nail cream strengthens the matrix or growing portion of nail which lies under the skin at base of nail. It can help prevent nail peeling and splitting. But it must be used faithfully for a period of time before a marked difference will be noted.

10. If polish becomes worn or chipped between manicures, remove it if you don't have time for repairs. Soft, weak nails will not hold polish as long as healthy ones.

NOTE: Your polish should match or harmonize with your lipstick.

Eye Care

It goes without saying that eye beauty basically requires 1) good eating and sleeping habits, and 2) corrected visual defects and ailments. What *does* need saying is that the eyes and the surrounding area should get only deluxe treatment.

Your eye is the most perfect, complex and most fragile of all your body organs. The slightest defect in its dimensions, its shape or its movements will cause trouble.

If you find your eyes become watery, irritated and burn—without apparent cause—cease using make-up, and get an examination.

If your eyes become irritated after long periods of use or because of temperature change, give them a bath. (You can use a warm extract of cornflowers or even tea, but anything containing collyrium should only be used with a physician's advice.)

If you find you need glasses, don't hestitate. Wear them. Glasses DO have an important beauty role. They can serve to strengthen a personality, help overcome timidity and give more assurance. The sentiment that: "men seldom make passes at girls who wear glasses" is passé. Today glasses can be fashionable as well as functional.

The use of glasses has solved a lot of nagging problems, such as constant headaches, nausea and dizzy spells. All it takes to find out if glasses are the solution to such problems is a visit to an oculist. If he prescribes glasses, get them. Be conscious about the frames. Just as the lenses are designed for your eyes, the frames should be made to fit the shape of your face, the arch of your brow and so on.

Eye troubles nowadays usually can be quickly detected and corrective procedures rapidly prescribed. Below is a description of the most common eye ailments.

A. *Myopia* or near-sightedness, is the most common of all eye ailments. People who suffer from myopia see whatever is close perfectly clear sometimes. In fact, at close range, they often see more exactingly than persons with normal vision. But, to see at a distance, they squint—a most unbeautiful and unbeautifying habit. Anything distant appears hazy to myopia sufferers and, by squinting, the light rays entering the eye are equalized, helping to clarify the outline of the distant object.

Myopia can be an advantage for certain types of precision work, such as clockmaking and jewelry work.

Since it is often hereditary, children of parents who have the condition should have their eyes examined at the earliest possible age.

The trouble might be slight, so it may be necessary to wear glasses only when seeing a movie, or in classes, or while doing anything which requires seeing distant objects.

If myopia is pronounced, glasses should be worn at all times to avoid further straining of the eyes. This condition, which generally becomes more pronounced during the formative and growing years, becomes stabilized in the early twenties. Myopia sufferers must realize that their eyes are particularly delicate and they should have periodic examinations—whether or not there is apparent cause for them.

B. *Hypermetropia* is commonly called "farsightedness" and it is the exact opposite of myopia. The eyes of the sufferers are smaller than normal, and objects which are near are out of focus, but distant objects may seem quite clear. As in myopia, corrective lenses are available.

C. *Astigmatism* may be associated with either myopia or hypermetropia, or it may be totally unique. In the astigmatic eye, the cornea—which is the anterior transparent part of the eye—has an unevenly rounded surface. Compensation for this can easily be made with special lenses. Astigmatism is fairly common and in many cases will pass unnoticed as long as it does not create more important troubles.

D. *Presbyopia* is a form of hypermetropia, but is not truly an eye defect. Rather, it is a normal transition which occurs around the age of forty-five or fifty.

At this period, the crystalline lens begins to lose its elasticity. The clarity of objects becomes lessened, particularly when they are close.

A balance must be made, and it would be senseless to avoid wearing glasses to read or sew without suffering. It is far better to wear glasses than to subject yourself to burning eyes and headaches.

If you are troubled with presbyopia, you should start wearing glasses with mildly corrective lenses and then every two or three years have the prescription rewritten.

Since in cases of presbyopia distant objects are clear while near objects are blurred, the corrective lenses are for clarifying the near objects. Naturally, it is annoying to have to put glasses on and take them off to accommodate the balance. The answer is double-duty glasses which have a small inset for close-range viewing. It takes time to become accustomed to glasses of this sort, but after wearing them a while, you will become accustomed to looking through the long range or close range portions of the lenses. In time, it will become automatic.

E. *Contact lenses:* If you're one of those women who stubbornly refuses to solve her eye problem with glasses, contacts may be the answer. The favored type of contact lens is the tiny one which fits over the cornea. These are so small and light they are practically invisible, but they have the same corrective values as ordinary types of glasses.

Contact lenses are usually prescribed for cases of myopia where the patient does not wish to wear glasses. The contact lenses thus have not only therapeutic value but also aesthetic value.

The wearing of these tiny vision aids is no problem— once the initial trial period has passed. But the fitting and making of them is most exacting.

Because of the close contact between the delicate cornea and a foreign material, there may be some minor discomfort and sometimes a slight irritation until the eye adjusts to this contact. But the discomfort is only temporary.

Remember: Persistent eye strain always calls for examination by an eye specialist. Always!

Occasional strain, however, can be relieved through compresses and bathing, as well as the eye bath previously mentioned.

A good compress can be made by soaking two wads of absorbent cotton in a mild solution of a teaspoon of boric acid to a glass of cool water. Just stretch out on your bed or couch, place the compresses over your closed eyes and rest for fifteen minutes.

A few drops of skin freshener in a glass of ice water is good for bathing your eyelids, temples and forehead.

Be gentle with the skin around your eyes. Handle it carefully. Don't squeeze, tug or pull it.

You can often help to keep crow's feet and wrinkles under control simply by applying a rich emollient cream on the areas where these unsightly conditions are prevalent.

Such a cream often contains lanolin and is often effective for lubricating.

Crow's feet, wrinkles and circles may sometimes be effectively concealed—but only temporarily—by applying a foundation base. Face powder that is lighter than your usual shade may also be helpful.

A good and quick "eye pick-me-up" is to apply hot and warm compresses alternately. You'll feel fresher immediately, but again only temporarily.

Pouches under the eyes sometimes call for treatment by an aesthetician.

Your own do-it-yourself eye treatments should begin by keeping the skin around your eyes as clean as possible. At night, apply a little oil to your lashes and brows. Brush them, and then apply an emollient cream to the area around your eyes. Be sure you get sufficient sleep and that your diet is a balanced one that includes foods rich in Vitamin A.

Ears

In spite of advanced methods, the talents of hair stylists are frequently strained in an attempt to deal with unsightly ears. If style decrees that hair shall be worn long and the ears covered then the problem is minimized. But female styles are fickle and sooner or later the fashion will be to have the ears exposed. This is the present trend and because of it the problem of ears arises. In previous centuries a woman's ears were as important to her beauty as were her mouth and her eyes, and she was proud to have them seen and admired. Perhaps evolution has, for some reason, caused ears to change, but it seems that they are no longer given much consideration in the scheme of beauty. However, their possibilities are still there. A delicate, shapely ear is still an emblem of femininity as much as a shapely nose, a full formed mouth, or lovely eyes. But, even knowing this, few women accord their ears more than passing attention. Explanation for this may lie in the fact that the human ear (contrary to those of most animals) is immobile and, in a sense, lifeless and without expressive value. We can develop a lively facial expression, smile, and so on, but the ears are stationary and inanimate. Even so, this is small reason for allowing them to detract from your beauty. They are visible and *can* be beautiful.

Ears should be well shaped and small; not so small as to appear absurd, but in keeping with the facial proportions. The best comparative measurements would be those of the nose and the ears. Ideally an ear should not be broader than the base of the nose, and in keeping with the length of the nose. This is, of course, taking into consideration that the nose itself is not malformed. Though the ears may be long, going a bit beyond the theoretic idea, they can still blend with a face which is fairly square and which has a pronounced jaw line. In such cases the various proportions compensate each other and give the effect of harmonious balance. If the ears do not meet the idealized requirements of beauty, so far as size is concerned, they can be cleverly masked with a large piece of jewelry or the arrangement of the hair.

More often than their size, it is the spread of the ears and their position in relation to the cranium that determines their aesthetic value. Ears should not stick out like flaps, nor should they lie flat against the head. They should not in any way detract from the balanced harmony of the face, or be remarkable as anything more than natural ornaments.

In my years as a beauty surgeon I have been visited by mothers asking that I perform corrective surgery on daughters of 4 to 5 years of age who have protruding ears. While this type ear may be indicative of a sympathetic, generous, honest and dynamic personality, on the aesthetic plane it can be the cause of psychological complexes. But such operations are *not* advised before the fifth year and in no case should a child be forced into it. One should never forget that, where beauty is concerned, a personal desire for amelioration is a primary factor. Any physical modifications which are not agreed to voluntarily can create emotional problems which are far more distressing than the existing physical ones. Among adults, during the past few years, corrective operations for this type of ear deformation have greatly increased, possibly because women find that protruding ears are an aesthetic handicap even when they are concealed by the hair.

In order to understand how ear defects can be corrected, it might be well to understand a little about the structure of the ear. The external ear acts as a sort of horn that captures sound and directs it into the inner ear; the part of the ear surrounding the opening to the inner ear is called the conch. The small protective flap which juts back, just over the inner ear canal, is the tragus, and from this extends a sort of fold in the ear, and this is the anthelix. Just above the ear lobe is another flap; the antitragus. The outer rim of the ear is the helix. Protruding ears are due to nothing more than a malformation of the anthelix, and the aesthetic surgeon, by reforming this fold, can bring the ears closer to the head. There are also other ear defects that can easily be corrected by slight alterations in the basic formations; large ears can be made smaller, spiney edges of the helix can be eliminated, a too large or too small tragus can be altered to more desirable proportions; even the ear lobes, if they are oversized, can be made smaller. But, should the lobes be too small, it is much more difficult to make them larger. No matter what, if the ears do not measure up to beauty standards, there is a corrective procedure.

External ear operations are quite simple and painless and are usually performed with a local anesthetic. But, though the operation may be benign, cautionary measures must be observed after the operation. After any ear operation the patient should rest for a few days and avoid any undue excitement. Corrective surgery of this type is most often undergone by young adults or adults, the greater number being among professional people who are constantly in the public eye. But there is yet another, and even larger group of women, who should and can make the most of their assets in order to be a beautiful mother, a beautiful wife, or simply a beautiful woman.

Part VII

Life Is a Glorious Adventure
—Try It!

The important thing in life is to have a great aim and to possess the aptitude and the perserverence to attain it.

—GOETHE

Part VII

Life is a Glorious Adventure
—Try It!

Do-It-Yourself Cosmetics

Beauty remedies have been used for thousands of years. The formulas, refined through the centuries, have been handed down to us. Centuries ago, the purpose of cosmetics was to enhance, to beautify, to cover up, to highlight. Today, the purpose is still the same. In this respect, woman is eternal. She always has desired to be beautiful, because beauty has always been desirable.

On the following pages you will find up-to-date formulas for making a whole variety of cosmetics right in your own home. These "beauty tools," plus any commercial beauty products which are personally satisfying to you, are some of the most important toys you'll use in "Playing the Beauty Game."

Try these suggestions. Make those products you need. See how satisfying it can be to have a "do-it-yourself" beauty laboratory right in your own kitchen.

One word of caution before you start. There are no preservatives in any of these cosmetics. Therefore, store the bulk of any you make in your refrigerator (along with any of the basic ingredients you have purchased to make them.) Keep only a small amount in containers on your dressing table. You can make enough to last a few weeks, but only put out enough to keep you going for a few days. Keep replenishing your dressing table containers. In this way, your do-it-yourself cosmetics will stay fresh and be as beneficial as possible.

All the ingredients for these cosmetics can be found in most drug or health food stores.

MEASUREMENT TABLE

1 oz. equals 31 grams
1 grain equals .065 grams
1 dram equals 4 grains
1 teaspoon equals 1 fluid dram
1 tablespoon equals ½ fluid ounce
1 teacup equals 4 fluid ounces

"Jet Set Special"

Make a pack of sea salt mixed with warm water until it is the consistency of moist sand. Before applying, it is better if you steam your face a little, or hold hot towels over it for a few minutes. You can leave the pack on for about fifteen minutes. If you want to give it the professional touch, put on the pack, then lie down and apply hot towels over the face.

The use of sea salt as a pack has been noted as a "remodeling massage". It has been said to "wipe off weariness and wrinkles". It will not only give your skin a lovely freshness, but the salt has a tightening effect—truly a "remodeling massage," while you do nothing.

Abstracting substances from the sea is now a serious venture for many products that are coming into general use in our daily lives. You can buy sea salt in all health food stores and in some drug and grocery stores.

"Debutante's Delight"

Beat the white of an egg until it peaks. Add one heaping teaspoonful of honey. Mix well.

Pat the masque on your face and neck (avoid eye area). Leave it on until you feel the drawing action (about five minutes). Wash off with cool water.

This preparation is a marvelous preliminary to your make-up for those special party-type occasions.

Remember the excess mixture keeps well for several days in your refrigerator. Before you reuse it, beat the mixture for about thirty seconds.

"Lover's Lotion"

2 tbs. lecithin
2 tbs. water
4 tbs. apricot kernel oil
a few drops of your favorite perfume

Blend until smooth.
Directions for use: Smooth gently on face and neck. It will be absorbed by the skin and leave a smooth velvety surface that will retain moisture.

This multi-purpose moisturizing cream, hand cream and make-up base is excellent for all three functions. You can apply make-up directly to your face over this preparation, or if used as a moisturizing facial cream, apply and allow your skin to absorb the beneficial ingredients. As a hand cream apply to hands as you would any other hand lotion.

"Garden of Eden Masque"

1 peeled cucumber
1 head lettuce (chopped)
1 peeled and chunked potato

2 slices lemon (rind included)
1 teaspoon dried peppermint leaves
1 teaspoon dried rose hips
1 teaspoon dried orange blossoms

Mix in blender.

Blend cucumber first. Wash lettuce. Add lettuce slowly with water that clings to leaves from washing. This will give just enough moisture to complete the blending. Add potato, lemon and herbs.

Place mixture on lettuce leaves and apply to face and neck. Over this apply hot towel. Steam in this manner for twenty minutes, reheating towel when necessary.

This fabulous herbal pack will make you feel as though you'd taken a fast trip to Paradise.

"Going Native"

1 tablespoon peppermint leaves
1 tablespoon eucalyptus leaves
1 teaspoon juniper berries
1 teaspoon chamomile tea
2 cups water

Bring all ingredients to a boil. Let them simmer for three minutes. Place mixture in open pan. Put a towel over your head and allow the vapor to steam your face and neck.

Of course, the pan can be eliminated if you have a vaporizer-humidifier. If so, follow instructors for its use.

"Eggs-Bees-Vee's Facial Pack"

(Pack for Ultra-Sensitive or Irritated Skins)
2 egg whites
2 teaspoons Tupelo honey (a mild and very delicate
    honey that can be obtained at a health food store)
1 tablespoon creamed papaya
1 capsule Vitamin E (oil type)

Beat egg whites until stiff. Add honey and creamed papaya (if you use fresh papaya be sure it is very ripe and mash it). Leave on face until drawing sensation is felt. Remove gently by dashing tepid water on the face. When skin is clean prick Vitamin E capsule, apply to face and neck and allow to remain on overnight. The Vitamin E capsule can be applied any night (without previously using the pack) as a healing night oil.

"Hot-Scotch" Facial

½ cup brewer's or nutritional yeast
½ cup scotch oatmeal
½ cup finely ground cashew nuts
2 teaspoons finely ground chili pequines
½ cup honey
3 egg whites

Blend in mechanical mixer or blender. Apply to face and neck. Allow to remain for ½ to ¾ hour. Wash face clean and apply cosmetic vinegar as in above recipe.

This masque cleanses the skin by increasing circulation. You will notice "flushing" or mild burning sensation. Those with extremely sensitive or allergic skins should eliminate the chili pequines from the recipe.

"East Indian Herbal Masque"

Take a quantity of bay leaves, add 1 cup of tea (freshly brewed), put ingredients in a blender until mixture is of the consistency to spread. Store this mixture in a dark place for 72 hours. The herbal masque is then ready to use for a relaxing facial.

"Queen's Delight Creme"
(Tired Skin Pick-Up)

1 teaspoon royal jelly honey
1 teaspoon water-soluble lecithin powder
1 teaspoon avocado oil

Mix thoroughly and apply to skin. Leave on for several hours —or overnight.

"Bye-Bye Blemishes"

For sunburns, cuts, burns, blemishes

¼ cup aloe vera gel (obtainable at your health food store under several different brand names)
1 tablespoon water-soluble lecithin powder.

Mix in blender. Apply and allow to remain on as long as possible, at least 15 minutes at a time, but preferably for several hours.

"Moon-Glow" Facial Sauna

Fill any kitchen pot with 2 quarts of water. Add a ripe lemon cut in half. Boil for 3 minutes. Add a heaping tablespoon of all or any of the following herbs: juniper berry, hibiscus, linden, peppermint. (These usually come packaged as herb teas.)

Place the pan on a table (with hot pad under it). Protect your hair with shower cap. Place large turkish towel over both your head and the pot and allow the deep penetrating steam to work for a good 3 to 4 minutes.

A good time to take the facial sauna is just before a shampoo—or the night before you shampoo. If taken at this time, do not use the shower cap and allow the penetrating steam to work into the scalp also.

"Super Shampoo" Rinse

(Acid Mantle Aide)

Whenever you shampoo your hair, wash your face or neck, or take a bath or shower, chances are you are destroying the protective acid mantle of your skin. Most soaps are destructive to Nature's "seal." To restore the acid balance, use a special vinegar made this way:

Into 1 pint of water, put ¼ cup dried peppermint leaves. Bring to a boil. Simmer for 5 minutes. Strain and add to 1 pint of apple cider vinegar.

This restorer should be used as a rinse when shampooing, as an astringent for the face and neck, and 1 cup can be added to the bath water.

"Sunny-Side Up Masque"

2 eggs
sweet cream

Mix egg whites with enough cream to make the preparation spreadable. Apply to thoroughly clean face and neck. Let liquid dry on skin for thirty minutes. Think happy thoughts. Wash face with tepid water. Rinse with cold water. Dry well.

"Milkmaid's Jewels Masque"

1 can powdered milk
4 tsp. tepid water ⎫ to paste
4 tsp. milk ⎰

Spread over face and neck—take a complexion brush and go over skin. When skin seems blush red, rinse off with tepid water. Reapply. Lie down for ten minutes. Cover eyes with saturated eye pads. Think of the serenity of a large cool farmhouse. Rinse off with lukewarm water. Rinse with cold water.

"Day Dreamer's" Bath

1 cup Epsom Salt
1 cup Baking Soda
1 cup sea salt
1/4 cup sulphur flowers (powdered)
10 drops of your favorite perfume

Use 1/2 cup in bath water. Relax. Daydream. Feel and look beautiful.

"Lime Tonic" Bath Oil

1 cup safflower oil
1 cup sunflower seed oil
1 tablespoon shampoo (free of detergent)
2 tablespoons lime extract

Mix in blender. Use about two tablespoons in bath tub. Allow water to run full force over oil.

"Rose Water—After Bath Splash"

Take 2 handfuls of scented red rose petals and put them in a jug or earthen pot. Pour over them 2 pints of water and 1/2 lb. sugar. Let them steep for 1 hour. Take the water and roses and pour them from one vessel into another until the water is scented with the flowers. Strain and keep in a cool place. Use this as a frequent "cologne-type" after bath splash to make yourself feel feminine all over.

"Ooh-La-La Paque"

1 teaspoon Fuller's Earth
2 teaspoons oat meal
1 teaspoon French chalk (talc)
1 teaspoon mentholated glycerine
6 drops tincture of benzoin

Mix with enough witch hazel so that it will spread easily. Allow pack to remain on your face for thirty to forty-five minutes. Remove with cold, wet towels.
This is a great facial pack for rejuvenating your skin.
For the same purpose, here is an alternate formula.

6 ozs. almond meal
3 ozs. Fuller's Earth
1 oz. tincture of benzoin

To these, add just enough witch hazel to form a thin paste. Apply on face and neck. Leave on for thirty to forty-five minutes. Remove with cold, wet towels.

"Sweet Dreams" Night Creme

4 ounces plain yogurt
6 tbs. lecithin (water dispersable only)
2 tbs. linseed oil (edible variety)
2 tbs. wheat germ oil
2 tbs. apricot kernel oil
1 tbs. avocado oil
1 tbs. sunflower seed oil
3 tbs. water
1 tbs. potato flour
5 drops of your favorite perfume

Mix all ingredients in blender until smooth. Apply to face and neck. Allow to remain overnight.

"Nuts to You"
(Dead Tissue Cleanser)

1 tablespoon almond meal (grind almonds very fine or use almond butter)
1 cup creamed papaya
1/4 cup lecithin powder (water dispersable only)
1/2 cup walnut oil

¼ cup wheat germ oil
1 tablespoon lemon extract

Mix all ingredients in blender until very smooth. Massage into skin thoroughly. Remove gently with tissues. Repeat several times. Papaya eats dead tissue while protecting the living. (Because of this fact papain, the active ingredient in papaya, is used as a meat tenderizer.) Fresh papaya can be used, but the best is the creamed, concentrated papaya. All these ingredients can be found easily at a health food store.

"Parisian Aromatic Bath"

Boil for 5 minutes, in a sufficient quantity of water, one or all of the following: bay leaves, thyme, rosemary, majoram and lavender. Strain. Add a small snifter of brandy. Shake the required quantity into a hot bath. Feel like Empress Josephine!

"Tropical Temptation" Bath Oil

1 cup sesame seed oil
¼ cup avocado oil
¼ cup apricot oil
1 cup cottonseed oil
1 tablespoon detergent-free shampoo
1 tbs. rose extract

Mix in blender. Start bath water. Add 3 tablespoons bath oil. Allow water to run full force over it.

"Roman Rose" Bath Oil

Fill a ceramic or pottery jar (do not use glass) with fresh rose petals. Pour a little olive oil over the petals. Store this mixture in the darkest place you can find in your home. Wait eight days and then retrieve your "Beauty Brew". Use the resultant sweet smelling oil to cleanse and beautify yourself. NOTE: You may substitute other flower petals for roses, as well as fragrant leaves, such as eucalyptus, or blossoms from a backyard citrus tree.

"Oil's Well That Ends Well"
(Hot oil shampoo)
Excellent aid for excessive dandruff or where hair is dry

and brittle, also especially helpful after too much exposure to sunshine.

1. Brush the hair and scalp.
2. Apply *warm* olive or castor oil to the scalp with cotton. Caution: Do not get oil hot enough to burn the scalp. Before you apply oil, you should apply heat to the scalp with hot towels wrung dry, or by use of a therapeutic lamp.
3. Massage oil into the scalp as thoroughly as possible with finger tips, as in shampooing. Leave on 15 minutes.
4. Shampoo through with warm water.

The hot oil shampoo may be done as often as every other day in severe cases of dandruff or dryness, but usually once a week is enough.

"Rosemary Hair Rinse"

Take a bunch of rosemary, cover it well with water and simmer for $1/_2$ hour or more. Strain. Use after shampoo. A delicate fragrance and a tonic effect is given to the hair when this preparation is used as your final rinse.

"Bittersweet" Facial Astringent

$1/_2$ cup apple cider vinegar
1 cup water
$1/_2$ cup cream of tartar
1 tablespoon lemon extract

Blend until smooth. This must be shaken each time it is used. Directions for use:
In the morning, gently wash eyes and ears with tepid water. Pat dry. Use astringent on face and neck for morning perk-up. Do not use soap or water on face and neck except very rarely.

Oily Skin Bracer

Ice applications stimulate circulation and help firm tissues. Take 3 or 4 ice cubes, put them into a thin towel and crack so ice is in bits. Dip towel in witch hazel. Go over face and neck with up-lifting motion. Keep this up for five minutes. Try to repeat this ritual at least three times a week.

A "Hint of Mint Masque"

2 egg yolks
1/2 cup safflower oil
1 1/4 tsp. mint extract

Beat egg yolks. Add safflower oil. When liquid begins to thicken, add mint. Blend well. When liquid is of thick enough consistency, spread it generously on face and neck area. Allow preparation to dry. Rinse off with tepid water. Rinse with cool water.

Basic Buttermilk Masque

This mask has only one ingredient—the buttermilk itself. As you familiarize yourself with this masque, the proper quantity will become apparent. Smooth buttermilk over the face and neck area. Let it dry. Rinse off—rubbing briskly with a wash cloth. Follow with a good, mild skin lotion.

NOTE: You can also use a quantity of oatmeal—moistened slightly— and receive the same beneficial results.

"Papaya Paque"

1/2 cup creamed papaya
1/2 cup almond oil
1/2 cup apricot kernel oil
1/4 cup water dispersable lecithin
1 tbs. castile or other shampoo (do not use a detergent
    base shampoo)
1 tbs. almond extract

Blend all ingredients together until smooth. Massage lightly over face and neck. Remove with tissue. Repeat twice more to remove all possible dead tissue and other make-up material so that the skin and pores can breathe.

This cleansing cream is especially effective because papaya attacks dead tissue while protecting the living ones. Natives of the South Seas have used papaya as a cosmetic for centuries. It is an effective cleanser for destroying those tiny, almost invisible particles of dead tissue on the skin. Any form of papaya may be used; the most effective is the creamed papaya which you will find in your local health food store.

Facial A La Creme

(To cleanse, soothe and stimulate)

3 teaspoons of almond meal
3 teaspoons of milk

Procedure: Remove make-up—cleanse skin thoroughly. Then apply mask over face. *Caution*: Do not allow mixture to get into eyes or nostrils. Remove paste with moistened towel. Sponge the face with warm milk. Follow with mild astringent.

Variation

(Using powdered *whole* milk)

Add three teaspoons of warm (not hot) water to three heaping teaspoons of the powdered *whole* milk. This will make a thin paste. First, wash your face and neck thoroughly. Then spread the paste over your face and neck in an even, thin coat. Next, take a complexion brush (or any small brush suitable for use on the face) and rub or brush the paste into the skin, right into the pores. As you do this, you will set up a slight irritation of the skin, which is highly beneficial. But do *not* overdo the brushing, especially at first. You will soon learn just how much brushing your skin can stand without excessive irritation.

After the skin is slightly blushed with color, rinse off the milk paste with warm water. Apply another coat. Allow this second coat to dry on your face and neck; let it get dry enough so that it rolls under the fingers like putty, but not enough to be powdery. This drying process is very important.

Now remove the film of rubberlike paste by rubbing it off with the tips of your fingers, much as you would remove a pencil mark from paper with an eraser. This removing process is also important. This should be done at night so the slight irritation or redness will be gone by morning. When you finish the treatment, do not apply any cream, powder, water or any other material to your face until the following morning.

Part VIII

Life Is Knowledge—Gain It!

Culture is to know the best that has been said and thought in the world.

—MATTHEW ARNOLD

Basic Beauty Encyclopaedia

CHAPTER THIRTY-ONE

A

Abrasion A broken place in the skin.

Acne A chronic inflammation of the sebaceous glands.

Adipose tissue Fatty tissue.

Aesthetics The laws and principles determining the beautiful in people, nature, art, etc.

Alcohol A votatile, inflammable, colorless liquid with a penetrating odor and burning taste—used as a germicide, and in conjunction with various beauty products.

Alkali Any caustic base, such as soda or potash, used in the making of soaps.

Almond Oil Kernels of bitter almond are bruised to obtain the oil which is used in the making of perfumes and soaps, most often in combination with lily of the valley.

Ambergris The most valuable and important fixative, known to be used as far back as the 15th century.

Ammonia A transparent, volatile gas, used to speed up the action of a bleach.

Antiseptic Any agent used to prevent the growth of bacteria.

Aroma A distinctive, agreeable fragrance or odor.

Assimilate To absorb or appropriate into the body.

Astringent A substance used to produce a contraction of the tissues.

B

Balsam Valuable as a fixative and note-giver in perfumes. The substance is obtained from tree barks by an intricate process. The bark is beaten and then covered with cloth which soaks up the liquid from the tree.

Basil The oil comes from the basilicum plant. When dried it is used as a spice in cooking. In the field of perfume it is used most often to enhance the violet fragrance.

Bath Oil Contains perfume concentrate in an oil base. Some bath oils are foaming; some make water feel softer in addition to perfuming the skin.

Beauty Culture The study of the improvement of appearance.

Benzoin A balsamic resin used as a stimulant and in perfumes.

Boric Acid Any acid derived from boric oxide. Used as an antiseptic chiefly for eye wash preparations.

Brilliantine A cosmetic preparation used to give highlights and gloss to the hair.

C

Calorie A unit of body heat used to measure food values.

Camomile An herb whose flowers are used in making hair and beauty preparations.

Capilliary A minute blood vessel.

Carbohydrate A substance, such as sugar, starch, cellulose, etc. composed of carbon, hydrogen, and oxygen.

Castile A Spanish province which gave its name to a good hard soap with olive oil.

Cell A minute mass of protoplasm forming the structural unit of every organized body.

Cholesterol A constituent of all animal fats. It is a natural product of the skin. The percentage of cholesterol in the skin determines the youthfulness. As we grow older the skin loses its cholesterol content, and in order to keep it supple it is advisable to use an agent which can be applied to the skin to replace the cholesterol and water that has been lost. This loss comes either through age or natural dehydration, due to exposure to the elements such as sunlight and weather. Any agent such as creams, lotions or other cosmetics containing cholesterol are beneficial. One of the principal sources of cholesterol is lanolin, which naturally contains 14% cholesterol.

Citric Acid Acid found in the lemon or orange.

Citrus Oils Oils used in perfumes, soaps, and most frequently in colognes to give a refreshing, perky note.

Cologne A perfumed toilet water.

Complexion General appearance of the skin, especially the face.

Corium The derma or true skin.

Cosmetic Therapy Any remedy, formula, or measure to beautify skin and body as a whole.

Cuticle The extremely thin outer layer of the skin or hair.

Cream Sachet A form of fragrance with a cream base which clings to the skin, making the scent last longer than a preparation with an alcohol base.

D

Dandruff A scalp dermatitis related to improper functioning of oil glands and often associated with excessively oily scalp. If a case of dandruff does not respond to a regimen of cleanliness with a special shampoo and stimulation, see your dermatologist or physician.

Depilatory An application for removing excess hair.

Derma Often called "the living skin", the derma consists of the underlayers of skin beneath the epidermis. There are very few cosmetics which either penetrate or alter the derma's functions. Beware of beauty products which claim to "feed" the underlayers of skin. The derma is kept healthy through the blood stream.

Dermatology The science which treats the skin and its diseases.

Diet A course of food selected with reference to a particular state of health.

Distillation A process in the making of perfumes where fresh blossoms are placed with water over wood fires and heated. The heat breaks open the cells, releasing the oil. The oil floats to the top and is separated. Nearly 4,000 pounds of roses are used to make one pound of rose oil.

E

Eau De Toilette Term used interchangeably with cologne. Both refer to a somewhat lighter form of fragrance than perfume, designed to be splashed on liberally. Used in combination with perfume, eau de toilette and cologne reinforce its fragrance and help create a lasting all over aura of scent. They are lighter and more fleeting when used alone.

Efficacious Having the power to produce the desired results.

Emollient A softening or smoothing agent which is relaxing and soothing to skin surfaces.

Emulsion In cosmetics, an emulsifying cream which has as its basis water and oil: i. e., mineral oil. A combination of liquids which do not dissolve into each other. The opposite of a liquifying cream.

Epidermis The cuticle or outer layer of the skin, actually composed of several thin layers. The epidermis is nature's protective covering for all human beings. Since it is the skin layer most affected by cosmetics, it should be properly cared for.

Essential Oil The essence, the intrinsic character, the necessary, unchangeable property of a specific fragrance. The essential oil of a flower possesses the best fragrance of that flower in a concentrated form. This is a volatile oil (evaporates unlike a fixed oil"). The vapors from a volatile oil stimulate the olfactory nerves, making us conscious of "odor". Essential oils are mainly obtained via steam distillation; when an extraction is made via use of fats or solvents, the resultant material is a *flower oil*.

Estrogen Estrogenic hormones (natural female hormones), when used in the amounts permitted by the Federal Food & Drug Authority are a helpful means of keeping a mature skin plump and youthful in appearance. When applied to the skin surface they do not affect internal organs. Useful only to the woman whose glandular system has slowed down in its own production of natural estrogen. Estrogen has been tested and used successfully in cosmetics for many years.

F

Falling Hair Each individual hair has a life span of about 180 days. It is then shed quite naturally and replaced by another. Excessively falling or thinning hair can result from dandruff or other scalp infection, from internal factors (such as pregnancy), or emotional strain and fatigue. These cases should be brought to the attention of a reputable physican.

Fatigue Body or mental exhaustion which can produce an acidity in muscle tissue and result in sagging.

Fixative That which fixes or sets. In perfume, the fixative's role is to prevent the volatile ingredients from evaporating too rapidly. It also regulates balance of evaporation. The fixative binds together all of a perfume's ingredients and fixes them. There are four substances obtained from the animal kingdom which have the greatest fixative value. They are used only in very expensive perfumes because of difficulty in their being obtained. They are CASTORIM (from the beaver); CIVET (Civet cat); MUSK (musk deer); AMBERGRIS (from the sperm whale).

Flaccid Flabby, sagging, as in "flaccid skin." Skin without tone.

Flaky Scalp Often called dandruff, which it isn't! The scalp regularly sloughs off the outer layers of the skin, but this sloughing should not be noticeable on a normal, healthy scalp. Excessive flaking is caused by dry scalp, improper rinsing during shampoo, or a run-down physical condition. Basic treatment: thorough shampooing and rinsing, with extra brushing to stimulate scalp and remove loose flakes present.

Follicle A small cavity or gland; the depression in the skin containing the hair root.

Fuller's Earth A soft, earthy substance frequently used as a basic ingredient in facial packs and beauty masks.

G

Geraniol A chemical substance frequently used in conjunction with rose oil to enhance the ultimate fragrance of perfumes and colognes.

Gland A secreting organ of the body.

Glycerine A sweet oily fluid used as an application for chapped skin.

Gum Gumy materials used in perfumes and colognes both for odor and fixative qualities.

H

Hangnail Skin partially torn loose at the side of a finger-nail.

Herbal This word describes those skin care formulas containing the essence of herb plants; also used advantageously in eye pads.

Herpes An inflammation of the nerve endings in the skin.

Herpes Simplex Fever blisters or cold sores.

Hexachlorophene Also known as G-11, an antiseptic solution that reduces odor causing bacteria. It is most helpful in combating skin infection.

Humectant A moistening agent that draws moisture from the air. It is found in many beauty preparations especially for dry and normal skins. Both honey and glycerine are humectants.

L

Lanolin Purified fat from sheep wool. A non-alkaline emulsifier used in many beauty preparations primarily to combat dryness and rough or chapped surface skin. Lanolin is the only commercial fatty substance which approximates the natural fats excreted by the sebaceous glands of the skin.

Liquefy To make liquid.

Lotion A liquid used for bathing the skin.

Luster Gloss or shine.

Lipid The generic term for a family of fatty substances: lecithin, leichol, lipids. They vary as to specific types, but all are necessary for the satin sheen of a healthy, lovely-to-look-at skin.

M

Manipulation The process of treating, working or operating with the hands, or by mechanical means, especially with skill.

Massage A manipulation of the body done by rubbing,

kneading, etc. To relax, increase metabolism, relieve tension and pain.

Metabolism The continuous process by which living cells or tissues undergo chemical change; a constant building up of living matter to effect growth and supply energy.

Milia Also known as whiteheads, small whitish nodules in the skin due to retension of sebum.

Muscle The peculiar tissue whose special function is to exert physical force. It consists of greatly elongated cells which contract when stimulated.

Medicated Creams There is a whole new crop of preparations devoted to dealing with acne and other problems associated with excessively oily skins. Some of them conceal blemishes without curing them. But even that is an improvement.

The new creams are based on a recent dermatological discovery; that most cases of acne can be cured, or at least helped, through the use of a skin-drying agent. This is a detergent, or a derivative of sulphur, in combination with a germicide, generally resorcinol or hexachlorophene. Anyway, the woman with a problem skin, or the teenager, now has a choice of all the cosmetics she needs available in medicated form for her own type of beauty treatment.

Moisturizers These are light emulsions of oil and water which are not rich in emollient qualities. They usually are preparations which can be worn under make-up. The majority are created to be completely compatible with your own skin's protective coating or "acid mantle". They can help to supplement an acid deficiency in the skin.

Masques These are applied over the face and throat to stimulate skin and tighten pores. There are three basic types:

1. *Smoothing masque.* Softens dry skin, helps counteract graininess and temporarily contracts pores.
2. *Stimulating masque.* Firms facial contours, tightens pores, works on improved circulation and gives a glow to the complexion.
3. *Medicated masque.* Mildly abrasive, this helps draw out impurities and dirt which clogs the pores, and is especially advantageous to those with an oily skin, or the oily-dry combination skin.

N

Nape The back part of the neck.

Nerve A whitish cord, made up of bundles of nerve fibre through which impulses are transmitted from the central nervous system.

Nutrition The taking in and assimilation of food through metabolism.

O

Ointment Medicated salve. An external remedy.

Organic Pertaining to substances derived from living organisms.

Orris Very much like the violet in scent, it is used in perfumes and cosmetics, and also as a fixative for both soap and lavender water.

Ozone A gas used as an antiseptic and oxidizing agent.

Oxygen A colorless, tasteless, odorless gas; chemically active element existing in large quantity in air and water.

P

Patchouli This is an East Indian mint and the leaves of the plant are dried and go through the distillation process. This famous musty scent was used in ancient days by being woven into shawls. It has the most intense fragrance of any plant.

Pedicure The care of the feet and nails.

Perfume From the Latin: per means "through"; fume means "smoke". Perfumes originally burned as incense offerings to gods. Perfume is the purest form of fragrance, a concentrated mixture of essences usually suspended in alcohol. It is the longest lasting form of fragrance—especially when applied to the pulse spots where the warmth of the body quickly develops it to the full beauty. Aside from the essential oils themselves, perfume is the strongest dissolution of the fragrant oils.

Peroxide An oxide with the highest amount of oxygen; used in bleaching.

Petrissage A kneading or pinching movement used in massage.

pH Factor This is a technical term used to measure the degree of acidity or alkalinity in anything. The surface of your skin, if it is normal, is slightly acid, with a "pH" of around 6. This invisible acid covering is called the ACID MANTLE. It is known that those cosmetic products which are closest in pH content to that of the normal skin are the most soothing and beneficial.

Polyunsaturates These are not "new ingredients" as such, but they have only recently been made chemically stable, thus permitting their use in cosmetics. They have long been recognized as natural components of a healthy, normal skin. Unlike some other skin components, they are not manufactured by the body, but are ordinarily supplied through certain fatty foods, such as walnut meats and some vegetable oils. Like vitamins normally supplied to the body through the diet, polyunsaturates must be replenished regularly. Dry skins show a deficiency in the amount of polyunsaturates found in what we call a "normal" skin. Creams with polyunsaturates are effective in supplying the skin with these essential elements.

Pores Tiny openings at the surface of the skin which become clogged or enlarged due to improper cleansing.

R

Rejuvenate To make young or vigorous again.

Rosewood An oil from which is derived an alcohol called LINALOOL which is used in making all fine perfumes.

Royal Jelly A term used to describe the food substance manufactured by the bees for the queen bee. This ingredient has received much publicity, but, as of this time, there is no recognized scientific data proving that Royal Jelly can live up to the claims made for it.

S

Saturate To cause to become completely penetrated or soaked. That which has absorbed all it can hold.

Sebaceous Glands The oil glands of the skin.

Seborrhea An abnormal secretion of the sebaceous glands.

Silicones Protective barriers which keep natural moisture in and ward off intrusion of incompatible outside elements. A silicone preparation can help guard your skin against the harshness and drying of water, sun, wind, etc.

Split Ends The result of mistreated hair. Excess sun, permanent waves, dye, bleaches or lack of brushing will contribute to dry, split hair ends. Split ends are best removed by a "razor cut". The use of a good hair cosmetic preparation with lanolin, plus a creme rinse, should help condition dry, damaged hair.

Spray Mist A modified version of eau de toilette, formulated for use in a spray applicator. Although any version of a fragrance requires time to develop to its full beauty, spray mist in particular does not indicate its true character immediately on spraying. It should be judged only after it has had an opportunity to develop with the heat of the body.

T

Tan Sunburn. Pigmentation of skin from exposure to the sun.

Tepid Neither hot nor cold; lukewarm.

Therapeutic Curative.

Tincture An alcoholic solution of medicinal substance.

Tissue Cream A nourishing cream composed of fats whose chemical composition most closely approximates that of the ideal, healthy skin. Also considered a lubricating cream.

Translucent The term used to describe face powder with minimal or no pigment that can be applied frequently without color build-up.

Trauma Bodily injury caused by violence; emotional shock with a sometimes lasting effect.

U

Unadulterated Pure, unmixed, not diluted.

Unguent A salve or ointment.

V

Vinegar A sour liquid containing acetic acid, frequently used as a hair rinse.

Vitamin A nitrogenous substance of which certain quantities are essential to the diet of man.

Volatile Easily evaporating; diffusing freely.

W

Wen A sebaceous cyst, usually on the scalp. Also a bruise or eruption on the skin surface.

Witch Hazel An astringent extract commonly used in various health and beauty preparations.

Epilogue

Life Is Learning To Play The Game

As we said at the beginning, life is a game . . . a game of chance. By now you should have discovered that "learning to play the game" is the secret of having a relatively happy and productive stay on this good earth.

In an age when men have landed on the moon and begun to probe the mysteries of other planets, we here on earth should have at least perfected a way of living which would bring us the most in peace and happiness and success.

Unfortunately, too often we go through life with burdens on our backs, and heavy hearts, unable to see and enjoy the wonders of just being alive!

The purpose of this book has been to show you some of the ways in which you can achieve lasting beauty—both within as well as without. . . . We cannot guarantee your life will be free of all problems. But we *have* shown you a way of life which CAN be devoid of despair and desperation.

If you have learned to "Play the Beauty Game" then surely you are one of the world's most fortunate people. Because it is only by learning to play the game that you can fully achieve your potentials.

Life is a game . . . a challenge . . . a battle . . . an obstacle course . . . Life is a mystery . . . the greatest gift . . . a potpourri of pleasures and pains. Life is indeed a glorious adventure if you have learned to play the game . . .

to meet the challenges . . . to win the battles . . . to hurdle the obstacles . . . to solve the mysteries . . .

Life can be really worth living if you have taken its gifts . . . if you have dipped into its pleasures . . . because in the process you will have learned how to become a more beautiful, lovable you—forever!

Robert Alan Franklyn, M.D.
The Beauty Pavilion
8760 Sunset Boulevard
Hollywood, California 90069